CASANDRA STONE

Baby Sleep Made Simple

Easy and proven tips to nurture infants into developing healthy sleep habits

This book was professionally typeset on Reedsy.
Find out more at reedsy.com

Contents

Introduction   1

1 Understanding Baby Sleep   5

The Science of Baby Sleep Cycles   5

How Baby Sleep Differs from Adult Sleep   8

Common Sleep Regressions and How to Handle Them   11

Understanding Sleep Associations and Their Impact   14

The Role of Circadian Rhythms in Infant Sleep   17

Developmental Changes and Their Effects on Sleep   19

The Importance of Naps and Daytime Sleep   22

Signs of Over-Tiredness and How to Avoid It   24

The Sleep-Feeding Relationship   27

Safe Sleep Practices to Prevent SIDS   30

2 Creating a Sleep-Friendly Environment   33

Setting Up the Perfect Sleep Space   33

The Role of Light and Darkness in Baby Sleep   35

Ideal Room Temperature and Humidity Levels   36

Using White Noise and Sound Machines Effectively   37

Safe and Comfortable Sleepwear   39

The Benefits of Swaddling and How to Do It Right   40

Managing Sleep Disruptions from External Noise   42

Creating a Consistent Sleep Routine   44

The Role of Naps in Maintaining a Consistent Routine   46

The Role of Comfort Objects and Loveys   47

Transitioning from Co-Sleeping to Independent Sleep   49

3 Gentle Sleep Training Methods   52

Understanding Gentle Sleep Training   52

The Pick-Up/Put-Down Method   55

The Chair Method: Gradual Removal Technique   57

The No Tears Method: Step-by-Step Guide   60

Establishing a Gentle Bedtime Routine   64

The Role of Parental Presence in Sleep Training   67

Gradual Night Weaning Techniques   70

Handling Sleep Disruptions During Training   73

Adjusting Sleep Training for Breastfed Babies   75

Troubleshooting Common Sleep Training Issues   78

4   Advanced Sleep Strategies and Solutions   82

Dealing with Early Morning Wake-Ups   82

Strategies for Short Naps   89

Sleep Solutions for High-Needs Babies   92

Managing Sleep During Illness   93

Transitioning to One Nap and Beyond   97

5   Parental Well-Being and Support   100

The Importance of Parental Sleep and Well-Being   100

Using Sleep Logs and Tracking Progress   102

Encouraging Patience and Persistence   104

6   Conclusion   107

7   Resources   110

Introduction

You've been awake for what feels like hours, rocking your baby back and forth, praying that this time, they'll fall asleep—and stay asleep. You've tried everything: singing lullabies, adjusting the room temperature, even tiptoeing out of the room only to hear them cry the second you close the door. You're exhausted, frustrated, and wondering if restful nights are ever going to be possible.

Sound familiar? You're not alone.

The truth is, sleep challenges are one of the most common struggles new parents face. And while there's no shortage of advice on the subject, the overwhelming information can leave you more confused than confident. That's where this book comes in. The purpose of this guide is to cut through the noise and provide you with practical, gentle sleep strategies that work—not just for your baby, but for your whole family.

This book was written to empower parents like you with the tools, strategies, and confidence to navigate baby sleep in a way that feels right for your family. You won't find rigid, one-size-fits-all methods here. Instead, we'll explore flexible, compassionate approaches that prioritize both your baby's emotional well-being and your peace of mind. Whether you're dealing with early morning wake-ups, multiple night wakings, or struggling with nap transitions, this book is designed to guide you through it all with patience and understanding.

As a parent myself, I know firsthand the sleepless nights, the tears (yours and theirs), and the overwhelming feeling that you're not sure if you're doing things "right." My own experiences navigating these challenges inspired me to create this book—a resource I wish I had when I was in your shoes. My motivation is simple: to help parents feel less alone, more supported, and better equipped to handle the ups and downs of baby sleep.

While there are countless books on sleep training, this one stands apart by offering a gentle, adaptable approach. You won't be asked to let your baby cry it out or follow strict schedules that don't align with your parenting style. Instead, this book focuses on understanding your baby's unique needs, working with their natural sleep patterns, and providing tools that foster trust and security. It's about creating a positive sleep environment for your baby, while also ensuring you get the rest and support you need.

Throughout the chapters, you'll find practical guidance on:

- Understanding the science behind baby sleep cycles and how they evolve as your baby grows.
- Creating a sleep-friendly environment that promotes longer, more restful sleep.
- Implementing gentle sleep training methods that are tailored to your baby's developmental stage.
- Addressing common sleep challenges, such as night wakings, short naps, and transitioning from two naps to one.
- Supporting your own well-being, because your sleep and mental health are just as important as your baby's.

Each chapter offers actionable steps and compassionate advice to guide you through the process.

You might be wondering, "Will this really work for my baby?" or "I've tried sleep training before, and it didn't help." It's important to understand that every baby is different, and what works for one child might not work for another. This book acknowledges those differences and offers a range of strategies, so you can find the one that feels right for your baby. And remember, sleep training isn't about instant success; it's a gradual process that takes time, patience, and consistency.

No parent should have to go through this journey alone. Throughout this book, you'll find reminders that seeking support—from your partner, family, friends, or even parenting communities—can make all the difference. Sharing your experiences with others who understand what you're going through can provide emotional relief and valuable insights. Parenthood is a team effort, and leaning on your community will help you stay strong and confident.

It's important to approach sleep training with realistic expectations. There will be progress, but there will also be setbacks—sick days, growth spurts, developmental milestones that temporarily disrupt sleep. That's okay. This book isn't about perfection; it's about making steady improvements and finding a rhythm that works for your baby and your family. Patience and flexibility are key, and the goal is to create a supportive environment that promotes healthy sleep habits over time.

As you begin this journey, I encourage you to embrace the process with an open mind and a gentle heart. Remember that every small step forward is a win, and you are doing an incredible job. If you're ready to create a sleep plan that works for both you and your baby, then let's get started—together.

Now, turn the page, and let's begin your path to better sleep for your whole family.

1

Understanding Baby Sleep

The Science of Baby Sleep Cycles

Understanding how babies sleep is one of the keys to helping them—and you—get more restful nights. Babies don't follow the same sleep patterns as adults. Their cycles are shorter, more fragmented, and focused on growth and development. By learning about the stages of baby sleep, how they evolve over time, and why it matters for sleep training, you can better anticipate your baby's needs and respond in ways that support their natural rhythms.

The Stages of Baby Sleep

Baby sleep consists of two main types: REM (Rapid Eye Movement) sleep and non-REM sleep, similar to adults but with key differences. During REM, babies are in a lighter sleep state where their brains are actively processing and developing, which is why this stage is vital for their cognitive growth. You may notice slight movements like twitching, smiling, or sucking during this phase, but because REM is so light, babies can wake up more easily.

Non-REM sleep is the deeper, more restorative part of the cycle, and it's divided into four stages:

1. **Stage 1**—Light sleep, during which the baby may still be easily woken. Their muscles start to relax, but they may still jerk or twitch.
2. **Stage 2** – A slightly deeper sleep where the baby's heart rate slows, body temperature drops, and their movements decrease.
3. **Stages 3 & 4** – The deepest stages of sleep where the baby is still, breathing steadily, and is least likely to wake. This is the most restorative part of the sleep cycle, supporting physical growth and recovery.

In contrast, adults spend much more time in non-REM sleep, particularly in the deeper stages, and far less time in REM sleep. This difference means that babies are more likely to wake frequently, especially in the first few months.

How Sleep Cycles Evolve as Babies Grow

Newborns have very short and frequent sleep cycles, usually lasting just an hour, with no clear distinction between day and night. This is why they wake so often—they cycle quickly through light and deep sleep, and the REM stage often rouses them.

Between 3 to 6 months, sleep cycles start to lengthen. Your baby will spend more time in the deeper stages of non-REM sleep, which means longer stretches of uninterrupted sleep, especially at night. By the time they reach 9-12 months, their cycles become more consistent and consolidated, helping them sleep for longer periods.

As your baby's sleep matures, naps may become fewer but longer, and they'll begin to establish a clearer day-night rhythm. Understanding these changes can help you adjust expectations and routines as your baby grows.

Why Understanding These Stages Matters for Sleep Training

Knowing your baby's sleep cycles is incredibly helpful when establishing sleep routines or attempting sleep training. Timing is key—intervening at the wrong moment can make things harder. For instance, trying to soothe a baby during REM sleep, when they are already more active, may result in more crying or fussiness.

Instead, recognizing when your baby is transitioning between stages can guide when to offer comfort or when to allow your baby to self-settle. You might notice that they briefly stir, shift, or make noise between cycles but may settle back to sleep on their own if given the chance. Timing sleep training interventions when your baby is in a deeper sleep stage will often be more effective.

Practical Tips for Observing Your Baby's Sleep Cycles

You don't need specialized equipment to get a sense of your baby's sleep cycles. Pay attention to their body language, movements, and breathing patterns. Here are some ways to track and observe their sleep stages:

- **Use of sleep trackers**: Some parents find technology helpful. There are various apps and devices designed to monitor your baby's sleep stages, though they're not always necessary.

- **Observing sleep patterns**: Notice when your baby is in lighter or deeper sleep. In lighter REM sleep, your baby may twitch, smile, or even briefly open their eyes. In deeper sleep, they will be very still, with slow, steady breathing.
- **Tracking behavior**: Keep a journal or note patterns. For instance, how long your baby sleeps between wake-ups, when they seem to be restless, and when they're in deep sleep. Over time, this will help you identify the natural rhythm of their sleep cycles, making it easier to plan naps and bedtime.

By learning these patterns, you'll be able to support your baby's sleep more effectively, reduce disruptions, and create a schedule that fits their natural needs.

How Baby Sleep Differs from Adult Sleep

If you've ever wondered why your baby's sleep patterns seem so different from your own, there's a good reason for it. Babies and adults don't just sleep for different lengths of time—they experience different sleep cycles. Understanding the physiological differences between baby and adult sleep helps explain why babies wake more often and why adult sleep solutions won't work for them.

Physiological Differences in Baby and Adult Sleep

One of the most significant differences between babies and adults is the amount of time spent in REM sleep. Babies spend roughly **50% of their sleep in REM** (Rapid Eye Movement) compared to only about 20-25% for adults. REM sleep is lighter, more active, and essential for brain development. It's when babies process the world around them, making it critical for learning and growth. However, since REM sleep is such a light stage, it also means that babies are more easily woken during this phase.

Another major difference is the **length of the sleep cycle**. An adult sleep cycle typically lasts about 90 minutes, including both REM and non-REM sleep stages, while an infant's cycle is much shorter—only 50-60 minutes. This shorter duration means that babies transition between lighter and deeper sleep more frequently, which is why they wake up more often. While adults can sleep for longer, uninterrupted stretches, babies naturally wake every 1-2 hours, especially in the early months.

Why These Differences Require Unique Sleep Strategies

Because baby sleep is structured differently, babies have **greater difficulty self-soothing**, especially in the early months. Their shorter sleep cycles and lighter REM stages mean that they wake frequently and often need help transitioning back to sleep. Trying to impose adult-like sleep expectations—such as sleeping through the night early on— can be frustrating for both parents and babies. Instead, baby-specific sleep strategies, like creating flexible schedules and responding to their natural sleep rhythms, are much more effective.

Debunking Common Myths About Baby Sleep

Many parents go into sleep training with misconceptions about what to expect. Let's clear up some common myths:

- **Myth: Babies should sleep through the night early on.** It's normal for babies to wake up frequently, especially during the first few months. Waking every few hours is a natural part of their development as they cycle through shorter REM and non-REM sleep stages. Expecting a baby to sleep through the night early on is unrealistic for most infants.

- **Myth: Longer daytime naps disrupt nighttime sleep.** Some parents worry that letting their baby nap too long during the day will prevent them from sleeping well at night. In reality, good daytime naps are essential for nighttime sleep. Over-tiredness from poor napping can actually lead to more wakefulness at night, not less.

Adapting to Baby's Sleep Needs

So, how can parents adapt to these differences? The key is to be flexible and responsive to your baby's unique sleep needs. Instead of following a rigid schedule, try these strategies:

- **Flexible sleep schedules**: Allow your baby to nap and sleep based on their natural rhythms rather than forcing them into a strict schedule. This might mean adjusting naptimes or bedtime based on how tired your baby seems. Flexibility helps ensure they get enough rest throughout the day and night.
- **Responsive parenting techniques**: Responding to your baby's sleep cues—such as yawning, rubbing their eyes, or becoming fussy—can help you put them to sleep before they become overtired. Recognizing and acting on these cues can lead to smoother sleep transitions and fewer nighttime wake-ups.

Being aware of the differences between baby and adult sleep and debunking common myths allows parents to set more realistic expectations and adjust their routines to support healthy, natural sleep for their baby.

Common Sleep Regressions and How to Handle Them

Sleep regressions can be one of the most challenging aspects of a baby's sleep journey. Just when it seems like you've established a solid sleep routine, your baby might suddenly begin waking frequently during the night or resisting naps. These phases are known as sleep regressions, and while they can be frustrating, they're a normal part of development. Understanding when they occur and why can help you better navigate them.

Common Stages of Sleep Regressions

There are several key times when sleep regressions are likely to happen, typically coinciding with important developmental stages:

- **4-month sleep regression**: This is one of the most well-known sleep regressions, often marking a permanent change in your baby's sleep patterns. Around this age, your baby's sleep cycle begins to mature, transitioning from the newborn sleep pattern into one that more closely resembles adult sleep, with distinct phases of light and deep sleep. This change can lead to frequent night wakings.
- **8-10 month sleep regression**: Around this time, babies are often hitting major physical milestones like crawling, pulling to stand, or even starting to walk. Their cognitive development is also rapidly advancing as they explore their environment more actively. These physical and cognitive changes can disrupt sleep as their brains process all these new skills.

- **18-month regression**: This sleep regression is often tied to another set of developmental changes, including separation anxiety, increased independence, and language development. It's also a time when toddlers may start resisting naps or bedtime as they test boundaries and express preferences.

Causes of Sleep Regressions

Sleep regressions are often triggered by developmental leaps or physical milestones. Here's what might be happening during these periods:

- **Cognitive leaps**: As your baby's brain develops and they learn new things—whether it's babbling, recognizing familiar faces, or mastering new skills like object permanence—it can disrupt sleep. Their brain is so busy processing all this new information that it can be difficult for them to settle down and sleep as they normally would.
- **Physical milestones**: Crawling, walking, standing, and even rolling over are exciting physical changes, but they can also cause sleep disruptions. Babies might practice these new skills in their sleep or wake up because they've moved into a position they can't easily get out of. Additionally, these new abilities can create restlessness or excitement that interrupts sleep.

Strategies for Managing Sleep Regressions

While sleep regressions can be tough, there are strategies to help manage them and keep both you and your baby on track:

- **Maintain a consistent bedtime routine**: Even though your baby's sleep might be disrupted, sticking to a predictable bedtime routine can provide comfort and help signal to your baby that it's time to wind down for sleep. Familiar cues like a bath, reading, or a calming song can be reassuring during periods of change.

- **Offer extra comfort and reassurance**: During regressions, babies often need a little more comfort than usual. Whether it's extra cuddles before bed, soothing words, or a quick reassurance if they wake during the night, being responsive to your baby's needs can help them feel secure, even during sleep disruptions.
- **Temporary adjustments to sleep schedules**: You might find that your baby needs a slightly different schedule during a regression. For example, they may require an earlier bedtime if they're waking up more frequently, or an extra nap if they're struggling to get through the day. Be flexible and adjust their sleep schedule temporarily to help them get the rest they need.

Reassurance and Realistic Expectations for Parents

It's important for parents to know that sleep regressions are **temporary**. While it can feel like your baby will never return to their usual sleep patterns, these phases do pass as your baby adjusts to their new skills and developmental changes. Encourage yourself to stay patient and persistent—regressions may last a few weeks, but with consistency and care, your baby's sleep will improve.

Remember that every baby is different, and some may experience sleep regressions more intensely than others. The key is to stay calm, provide comfort, and keep your expectations realistic. Sleep regressions are a normal part of growth and development, and with the right strategies, you can navigate through them successfully.

Understanding Sleep Associations and Their Impact

Sleep associations play a significant role in how babies fall asleep and stay asleep. Simply put, a sleep association is anything a baby has come to rely on to help them transition from wakefulness to sleep. These associations can either help or hinder a baby's sleep, depending on what they are and how they are used.

What Are Sleep Associations?

Sleep associations are the conditions or habits that a baby links to falling asleep. For example, if a baby is always rocked to sleep or fed before bed, they may come to rely on these actions to fall asleep each time they wake up. While these associations can seem harmless at first, they can cause issues if a baby is unable to self-soothe when they wake during the night.

Examples of common sleep associations include:

- **Rocking to sleep**: A parent rocks the baby to sleep, and the baby comes to expect this action to fall asleep.
- **Feeding to sleep**: The baby associates nursing or bottle feeding with falling asleep and struggles to sleep without it.
- **Pacifier use**: The baby needs a pacifier to fall asleep and wakes up when it falls out, unable to settle back down without it.

Positive vs. Negative Sleep Associations

Not all sleep associations are created equal. Some associations are **positive**, encouraging independent sleep and self-soothing, while others are **negative**, causing babies to rely on external help to fall asleep.

Positive sleep associations: These are the associations that allow a baby to fall asleep without external assistance. Examples include:

- **A lovey (comfort item)**: A small blanket or stuffed animal can provide comfort without needing a parent's intervention.
- **White noise**: A steady, soothing sound that helps drown out distractions and can play continuously throughout the night.
- **A dark, quiet room**: Creating an environment conducive to sleep can help the baby feel secure and relaxed, encouraging self-soothing.

Negative sleep associations: These habits require a parent or external factor to help the baby sleep. Examples include:

- **Needing to be held**: If a baby always needs to be held to sleep, they'll wake during the night and need the same level of assistance to go back to sleep.
- **Feeding or rocking**: While soothing, these actions can make it difficult for a baby to learn to sleep independently, as they rely on these actions to settle.

Strategies to Change or Break Negative Sleep Associations

If your baby has developed negative sleep associations, don't worry—there are gentle, effective ways to help them transition to positive ones. Here are a few key strategies:

- **Gradual fading techniques**: This method involves slowly reducing the amount of support you provide to help your baby fall asleep. For example, if you rock your baby to sleep, you could gradually reduce the amount of rocking over several days or weeks until they can fall asleep with less help. This gradual approach makes the transition smoother and less stressful for both baby and parents.

- **Introducing new sleep cues**: Along with fading out old habits, it's helpful to introduce positive sleep cues that encourage independent sleep. These can include a bedtime routine, a comfort item (like a lovey), or the sound of white noise. The goal is to create associations that your baby can control, rather than relying on your presence to fall back asleep.

Long-Term Benefits of Healthy Sleep Associations

Establishing healthy sleep associations early on can significantly improve your baby's sleep and overall development. By encouraging **self-soothing abilities**, your baby can transition between sleep cycles with less help, leading to fewer nighttime wakings. Babies who can self-soothe are more likely to sleep for longer, uninterrupted stretches, which benefits their well-being and yours.

Additionally, **independent sleep** fosters confidence and security as your baby grows. They learn to associate bedtime with calm, consistent routines that allow them to relax and drift off without needing outside assistance. This independence also helps as they move through different stages of development, making future sleep transitions smoother.

By breaking negative sleep associations and fostering positive ones, you're setting your baby up for a lifetime of healthy sleep habits, which will benefit them as they grow into childhood and beyond.

The Role of Circadian Rhythms in Infant Sleep

Understanding circadian rhythms and their role in infant sleep is crucial for establishing healthy sleep patterns. These biological processes regulate the sleep-wake cycle and gradually align with environmental cues like light and dark as your baby grows.

What Are Circadian Rhythms?

- **Biological Clock Regulation**: Circadian rhythms are natural, internal processes that follow a 24-hour cycle. They regulate the timing of sleep, wakefulness, and other physiological functions. These rhythms are heavily influenced by external factors, primarily light and darkness.
- **Influence on Sleep-Wake Cycles**: In adults, circadian rhythms signal the body when to feel awake and when to feel sleepy. For babies, these rhythms take time to develop, but they eventually help them differentiate between day and night, playing a vital role in sleep patterns.

How Circadian Rhythms Develop in Infants

1. **Initial Absence of a Circadian Rhythm**: Newborns are not born with fully developed circadian rhythms. For the first few months, their sleep-wake cycles are irregular, driven mostly by hunger and discomfort rather than the time of day.
2. **Gradual Alignment with Day-Night Cycles**: Babies begin to develop their circadian rhythms between 2 to 4 months of age, aligning more closely with the natural day-night cycle. As this biological clock matures, babies start consolidating their sleep

during the night and becoming more alert during the day.

Tips for Supporting the Development of Healthy Circadian Rhythms

Exposure to Natural Light During the Day:

Daytime Brightness: Ensure your baby gets exposure to natural light, especially in the morning. Natural light helps signal to their developing circadian rhythm that it's daytime, encouraging wakefulness during the day and sleepiness at night.

Consistent Bedtime and Wake-Up Times:

- **Predictable Schedule**: Establish a consistent bedtime and wake-up time to help reinforce your baby's developing circadian rhythm. Consistency sends a clear message to their internal clock about when it's time to sleep and wake.
- **Bedtime Routines**: Engaging in a calming pre-bedtime routine helps signal to your baby's circadian rhythm that nighttime is approaching, encouraging sleep.

Impact of Disrupted Circadian Rhythms

1. **Increased Night Wakings**: If your baby's circadian rhythm is not well-established or becomes disrupted, they are more likely to experience frequent night wakings. This can happen due to irregular nap schedules, lack of consistent exposure to natural light, or inconsistent bedtime routines.
2. **Difficulty in Establishing a Sleep Routine**: Without a well-regulated circadian rhythm, it becomes harder for your baby to

settle into a regular sleep schedule. This can lead to fragmented sleep and make it challenging to establish a reliable routine.

Supporting the development of your baby's circadian rhythm through exposure to light, consistent sleep schedules, and a predictable routine can help foster better sleep and smoother transitions between day and night. This natural alignment with their biological clock is key to creating lasting, healthy sleep habits.

Developmental Changes and Their Effects on Sleep

As babies grow, they experience several developmental milestones that can temporarily disrupt their sleep patterns. These changes, though exciting and a sign of your baby's progress, can often lead to more frequent night wakings or difficulty settling. Understanding how these developmental leaps affect sleep can help you navigate these temporary setbacks with greater confidence.

Key Developmental Milestones That Impact Sleep

Certain developmental milestones are more likely to affect your baby's sleep than others. These milestones often coincide with increased mobility, physical discomfort, or cognitive leaps, all of which can lead to sleep disruptions. The most common milestones that impact sleep include:

- **Rolling over**: Around 3-6 months, many babies begin to roll over, which can interfere with their sleep. Babies may roll onto their stomachs during sleep and struggle to roll back, leading to frustration and waking.

- **Sitting up**: Between 6-8 months, babies may start to sit up on their own. While exciting, this new ability can make it harder for babies to settle down to sleep, as they may sit up involuntarily during the night and need help lying back down.
- **Teething**: Teething can begin as early as 4-7 months and can cause significant discomfort, which often disrupts sleep. The pain and soreness from new teeth breaking through can make it harder for babies to fall asleep and stay asleep.

Connection Between Developmental Changes and Sleep Patterns

These developmental milestones often coincide with temporary changes in your baby's sleep patterns. Here's how specific milestones can impact sleep:

- **Increased mobility leading to frequent wake-ups**: As babies learn to roll over, sit up, and eventually crawl or stand, their newfound mobility can cause them to wake more frequently. They may roll into uncomfortable positions, or their curiosity to explore their new skills may keep them awake longer than usual.
- **Discomfort from teething**: Teething pain can disrupt both naps and nighttime sleep. The discomfort may make it harder for babies to settle down or cause them to wake up more frequently during the night, seeking comfort.

Strategies for Managing Sleep During Developmental Changes

Although these disruptions can be frustrating, there are ways to manage your baby's sleep during periods of developmental growth. The key is to offer support while maintaining as much consistency as possible.

- **Extra comfort during teething**: If your baby is teething, providing extra comfort can help ease the pain. You might offer a cool teething ring before bedtime or gently rub their gums. Over-the-counter teething gels or pain relief (with your doctor's approval) can also help minimize discomfort, allowing your baby to sleep more peacefully.
- **Safe sleep environment for increased mobility**: As your baby becomes more mobile, ensure their sleep environment is safe. This includes using a firm mattress in the crib without soft bedding, keeping the crib free from toys, and lowering the mattress height if your baby can pull themselves up. Also, offer plenty of opportunities during the day for your baby to practice their new skills, helping to release energy and build confidence, which may reduce nighttime disruptions.

Reassurance for Parents: These Changes Are Temporary

While developmental changes can lead to temporary sleep setbacks, it's important to remember that these phases are usually short-lived. Your baby's sleep will likely return to normal as they adjust to their new abilities or overcome the discomfort caused by teething.

The most effective approach during these periods is to remain **consistent with routines**. Stick to your usual bedtime routine as much as possible, and offer extra comfort and reassurance when needed. By maintaining predictability in your baby's day, you'll help them feel secure and more easily transition through these developmental milestones.

The Importance of Naps and Daytime Sleep

Naps are not just an opportunity for parents to get a break— they play a crucial role in a baby's overall sleep health and development. Daytime naps are essential for promoting better nighttime sleep and ensuring that your baby's cognitive, emotional, and physical development progresses smoothly.

The Role of Naps in Overall Sleep Health

Napping during the day is deeply interconnected with nighttime sleep quality. When babies don't get enough daytime rest, they can become overtired, leading to increased difficulty falling asleep at night, more frequent night wakings, and shorter sleep durations. On the other hand, well-rested babies who nap appropriately during the day are often able to settle into nighttime sleep more easily and sleep for longer stretches.

Naps also serve important developmental functions:

- **Cognitive and physical benefits of napping**: Daytime sleep helps babies process and consolidate what they've learned, making naps essential for brain development. Naps also support physical growth, especially during periods of rapid change, such as when a baby is learning to sit, crawl, or walk.

Optimal Nap Schedules by Age

As your baby grows, their nap needs will change. Understanding these changes and adapting your baby's nap schedule accordingly can help promote better rest and development.

- **Newborn nap schedules**: Newborns have shorter sleep cycles and spend a lot of time in REM sleep, which means they need frequent naps throughout the day. Most newborns nap about 3-5 times daily, with each nap lasting anywhere from 30 minutes to 2 hours.
- **Infant nap schedules (3-6 months)**: By 3 months, babies usually begin to establish a more regular sleep schedule. At this stage, babies typically take 3 naps a day— one in the morning, one around midday, and one in the afternoon. Each nap should last about 1-2 hours.
- **Infant nap schedules (6-12 months)**: Between 6-12 months, many babies drop the third nap and settle into a two-nap routine. These naps often occur in the morning and afternoon, each lasting 1-2 hours. As your baby nears their first birthday, naps may consolidate and lengthen, especially if they're getting adequate nighttime sleep.

Creating a Nap-Friendly Environment

A nap-friendly environment can make all the difference when it comes to ensuring your baby gets restful, rejuvenating sleep during the day. Here are some simple, actionable tips for creating a space conducive to napping:

- **Darkened room**: Keeping the room dark helps signal to your baby that it's time to sleep. Blackout curtains or blinds can be useful for creating a darker environment, especially during daytime naps.
- **Consistent nap location**: Ideally, your baby should nap in the same space where they sleep at night. This consistency helps them associate the environment with rest, making it easier for them to settle down and fall asleep.

Maintaining a consistent routine around naps— just like you would for bedtime— helps your baby recognize that it's time for rest.

Handling Nap Transitions

As babies grow and their sleep needs change, they'll naturally transition to fewer naps. While each baby is different, there are some general signs that it may be time to drop a nap:

- **Signs that it's time to drop a nap**: Your baby may show signs of being ready to drop a nap when they consistently refuse one of their naps or when they struggle to fall asleep at their usual nap time. Another common sign is when naps start cutting into their nighttime sleep, resulting in later bedtimes or early morning wake-ups.
- **Gradual transition strategies**: When it's time to drop a nap, do so gradually. You might start by slightly reducing the length of one of their naps, or by stretching their awake times between naps. This helps your baby adjust to the change without becoming overtired.

For example, when transitioning from three to two naps, gradually lengthen the time between the first and second naps until your baby can comfortably make it to the afternoon without needing a third nap. This transition period may take a week or two, but staying consistent will help smooth the process.

Signs of Over-Tiredness and How to Avoid It

One of the key challenges in maintaining a healthy sleep routine for your baby is recognizing and preventing overtiredness. When a baby becomes overtired, their ability to fall asleep and stay asleep becomes compromised, creating a cycle of disrupted rest. Learning to spot the early signs of tiredness and responding promptly is crucial for ensuring your baby remains well-rested and able to settle into restorative sleep.

Identifying the Signs of an Overtired Baby

Overtiredness can quickly lead to a baby becoming fussy and unsettled, making it more difficult for them to relax and fall asleep. Here are some of the most common signs that your baby is overtired:

- **Fussiness and irritability**: An overtired baby often becomes more fussy and cranky than usual. You may notice them crying more frequently or becoming irritable for no apparent reason.
- **Difficulty falling asleep**: Despite being tired, overtired babies can struggle to settle down and fall asleep. Their overstimulation can make it hard for them to relax, causing frustration for both the baby and the parent.
- **Shorter sleep duration**: When overtired, babies may not sleep as long or as deeply as they usually do. They may wake up after short periods of sleep and be unable to stay asleep for a full cycle.

The Consequences of Over-Tiredness

Overtiredness doesn't just affect your baby's mood— it can also lead to more significant disruptions in their sleep and overall well-being. The longer a baby stays overtired, the harder it can be to break the cycle of poor sleep.

- **Increased night wakings**: Babies who are overtired are more likely to wake up multiple times throughout the night. Their bodies have a harder time staying asleep, making frequent wake-ups common.

- **Difficulty in settling down**: Once overtired, it becomes much harder for babies to calm themselves. This makes bedtime more stressful, and getting them to settle for naps or nighttime sleep may take much longer.

Preventing Overtiredness

The best way to manage overtiredness is to prevent it before it begins. Here are some strategies that can help keep your baby well-rested and in a good sleep rhythm:

- **Recognizing and responding to sleep cues**: One of the most effective ways to prevent overtiredness is to pay close attention to your baby's natural sleep cues. These cues include rubbing their eyes, yawning, or becoming less engaged with their surroundings. As soon as you notice these signs, it's a good time to initiate a nap or begin the bedtime routine.
- **Maintaining a consistent sleep schedule**: Establishing a regular sleep schedule is key to preventing overtiredness. Predictable nap times and bedtimes help regulate your baby's internal clock, making it easier for them to fall asleep before they reach the overtired stage.

Helping an Overtired Baby Settle Down

If your baby has already become overtired, don't worry— there are steps you can take to help them calm down and get back on track.

- **Extra soothing techniques**: When a baby is overtired, they often need additional comfort to relax. Try using gentle rocking, swaddling (if appropriate for their age), or soothing sounds like white noise to create a calming environment. Skin-to-skin contact can also help provide extra reassurance.

- **Adjusting the sleep schedule temporarily**: If overtiredness has disrupted your baby's sleep routine, consider temporarily adjusting their schedule to allow for more frequent naps or an earlier bedtime. Short naps can help reset your baby's energy levels and prevent further overtiredness.

By taking proactive steps to prevent and manage overtiredness, you can help ensure that your baby remains well-rested and develops healthy sleep habits.

The Sleep-Feeding Relationship

The relationship between feeding and sleep is critical to understand as it directly influences your baby's rest. How and when your baby is fed plays a significant role in shaping their sleep patterns, especially during the first year. By establishing a balanced feeding routine, parents can help promote longer, more restful sleep periods and ease the transition into a more structured sleep schedule.

How Feeding Affects Sleep

The timing, frequency, and type of feeding can all have an impact on your baby's sleep. Night feedings, in particular, are closely linked to the sleep-wake cycle during the early months of life.

- **Impact of night feedings**: In the early weeks and months, babies often wake up frequently for night feedings due to their small stomach size and high metabolic needs. These night feedings are a natural part of their development, and as babies grow, the need for night feedings gradually decreases.

- **Role of full feedings in promoting longer sleep**: Ensuring that your baby has a full, satisfying feeding can help them sleep longer stretches. When babies receive complete feedings, especially before bedtime, they are more likely to stay asleep for an extended period rather than waking up due to hunger.

Feeding Schedules That Support Sleep

Creating a consistent feeding schedule that aligns with your baby's sleep needs can help foster better sleep habits. These schedules will evolve as your baby grows and their feeding requirements change.

- **Newborn feeding schedules**: In the early months, newborns typically need to eat every 2 to 3 hours, around the clock. This frequent feeding schedule is necessary to support their rapid growth and development, but it also means that sleep will be fragmented.
- **Adjusting feeding schedules as the baby grows**: As babies grow and their stomach capacity increases, the frequency of feedings decreases. By 3 to 6 months, many babies can go longer stretches between feedings, and by 6 to 12 months, some may be able to sleep for longer periods at night with fewer or no night feedings.

Differences Between Breastfed and Formula-Fed Babies

The method of feeding—whether breastfeeding or formula feeding— also influences sleep patterns. Each feeding method has its own set of dynamics that affect how long a baby can go between feedings and how long they might sleep.

- **Frequency of feedings for breastfed babies**: Breastfed babies tend to feed more frequently than formula-fed babies. Breast milk is digested more quickly, which often leads to shorter intervals between feedings, especially during the first few months.
- **Longer sleep stretches for formula-fed babies**: Formula-fed babies may sleep longer stretches at night because formula takes longer to digest, keeping them full for a longer time. However, it's important to note that every baby is different, and feeding method alone doesn't determine sleep habits.

Managing Night Feedings

Night feedings are a significant part of infant sleep in the early months, but as babies grow, parents often look for ways to reduce or eliminate these night feedings. Here are some strategies to manage and eventually minimize night feedings:

- **Dream feeding techniques**: A dream feed is a feeding that occurs right before the parent goes to bed, usually without fully waking the baby. The goal is to top off your baby's hunger before the longest sleep stretch, ideally helping them sleep longer during the night.
- **Gradual night weaning methods**: As your baby gets older and can take in more calories during the day, you can start gradually weaning them off night feedings. This can be done by slowly reducing the amount of milk offered during night feedings or gradually pushing back the time of the feeding until your baby is able to sleep through the night without needing to eat.

By understanding how feeding routines interact with sleep and adjusting them as your baby grows, parents can create a balanced approach that encourages better sleep habits over time.

Safe Sleep Practices to Prevent SIDS

Safe sleep practices are essential for reducing the risk of Sudden Infant Death Syndrome (SIDS) and other sleep-related infant deaths. By following established safe sleep guidelines, parents and caregivers can significantly decrease the likelihood of these tragic occurrences, ensuring that their baby sleeps in the safest environment possible.

Importance of Safe Sleep Practices

Following safe sleep guidelines is a proactive step in protecting your baby during sleep. Research has shown that adhering to these practices can reduce the risk of SIDS, which most commonly affects infants under 1 year old.

- **Back-to-sleep position**: Always place your baby on their back to sleep, both for naps and at night. This is the most effective way to reduce the risk of SIDS, as studies have shown that stomach or side sleeping increases the risk.
- **Safe crib environment**: A safe sleep environment extends beyond positioning. The crib or bassinet itself should meet safety standards, and extra care must be taken to avoid hazards like suffocation or entrapment.

Comprehensive Safe Sleep Guidelines

Creating a safe sleep space involves more than just positioning your baby on their back. These guidelines will help you ensure that your baby's sleep environment is as safe as possible.

- **Use of a firm mattress**: The mattress in your baby's crib should be firm and fit snugly within the crib frame. Avoid using soft mattresses, cushions, or pillows, as they can increase the risk of suffocation.
- **Avoiding loose bedding and soft objects**: Keep the crib free of loose blankets, pillows, stuffed animals, and bumpers, which can obstruct your baby's airway or cause entrapment. If additional warmth is needed, use a sleep sack or wearable blanket designed for infants.
- **Room-sharing without bed-sharing**: If you choose to share a room with your baby, but not the same bed. Keeping the baby's sleep space close to you can reduce SIDS risk and make nighttime care easier, but co-sleeping in the same bed can increase the risk of accidental suffocation or falls.
- **Maintaining a comfortable room temperature**: Avoid overheating your baby by keeping the room at a comfortable temperature. Overbundling or allowing the room to become too warm can increase the risk of SIDS.

Additional Resources for Safe Sleep Information

For further guidance on creating a safe sleep environment, parents can refer to expert recommendations and resources provided by trusted organizations. Here are a few reliable sources:

- **Pediatric guidelines**: The American Academy of Pediatrics (AAP) offers comprehensive safe sleep recommendations that include guidance on sleep positions, safe sleep environments, and strategies to reduce the risk of SIDS.
- **SIDS prevention organizations**: Organizations such as the

National Institute of Child Health and Human Development (NICHD) and First Candle provide detailed resources and support for parents looking to learn more about safe sleep practices and SIDS prevention.

2

Creating a Sleep-Friendly Environment

Setting Up the Perfect Sleep Space

Creating a safe and comfortable sleep space is foundational to promoting healthy sleep habits in your baby. By focusing on the essentials and eliminating unnecessary items, you can provide a soothing environment that encourages restful, uninterrupted sleep.

Essentials of a Safe and Comfortable Sleep Space

To ensure your baby's sleep area meets safety standards and provides maximum comfort, certain elements are non-negotiable. The first and most important component is a **firm, flat mattress**. The mattress should be designed specifically for a crib or bassinet and offer firm support. Soft mattresses or surfaces that contour to the baby's shape are not recommended, as they pose suffocation risks. The **crib sheet** should be snugly fitted around the mattress to prevent bunching, ensuring a smooth, flat surface for your baby to sleep on.

Additionally, temperature control is key. While it's important to keep your baby warm, the sleep space should not be too hot. Consider dressing your baby in appropriate layers of clothing rather than using blankets, which can lead to overheating and are not safe in the crib.

The Importance of a Clutter-Free Crib

A clutter-free crib is essential for both safety and promoting undisturbed sleep. Items like stuffed animals, pillows, loose blankets, and bumper pads can increase the risk of suffocation and entrapment, making the sleep space hazardous. Keeping the crib clear of these objects not only enhances safety but also reduces overstimulation, which is important for helping your baby relax and settle into sleep.

A simple, clean sleep space with minimal distractions supports a healthy sleep environment. When babies have fewer visual or tactile distractions, they're more likely to associate their sleep area with rest, helping establish consistent sleep patterns.

Choosing the Right Crib or Bassinet

Selecting a safe crib or bassinet is a critical part of setting up your baby's sleep space. When shopping for a crib, always look for **safety certifications** that ensure the product meets current standards. The crib or bassinet should be sturdy, with well-spaced slats and no risk of gaps where the baby's limbs could become trapped.

Size is also an important consideration. Ensure that the crib or bassinet is appropriately sized for your baby's age. Some bassinets are designed for newborns but will need to be transitioned to a crib as your baby grows, especially once they start rolling over or sitting up.

Arranging the Sleep Space Within the Room

The placement of your baby's crib or bassinet within the room also affects their safety and sleep quality. It's important to position the crib **away from windows, cords, and blinds** to prevent accidents and eliminate drafts. Additionally, avoid placing the crib near radiators or vents, which could cause your baby to become too hot or too cold during sleep.

Many parents opt to keep the crib or bassinet **close to their bed** for easier access during nighttime feedings or care. Room-sharing is recommended for the first six to twelve months, as it can help reduce the risk of SIDS while making it more convenient for parents to tend to their baby during the night.

The Role of Light and Darkness in Baby Sleep

Light plays a significant role in regulating a baby's sleep by influencing melatonin production, a hormone essential for sleep. Exposure to natural light during the day helps align a baby's internal clock, promoting healthier sleep patterns and reducing nighttime wakefulness. It's important to avoid screen time and exposure to bright artificial light in the hours leading up to bedtime, as it can interfere with melatonin production, making it harder for babies to settle down.

To create an optimal dark sleep environment, using blackout curtains can block out external light, making it easier for babies to fall and stay asleep. Reducing light from electronic devices like baby monitors or clocks is also crucial to maintain the darkness needed for uninterrupted sleep.

Nightlights can be helpful, but it's important to choose dim lights, preferably in red or amber hues, which are less likely to disrupt sleep. Nightlights should be placed away from the crib to provide just enough illumination for nighttime feedings or diaper changes without overstimulating the baby.

For naps during the day, managing light exposure is equally important. Using temporary blackout solutions, such as portable curtains for travel, can help ensure that a baby's sleep isn't disturbed by bright daylight. As babies grow older, sleep masks can also be introduced for naps, especially in unfamiliar environments or while traveling, to ensure consistent rest.

Ideal Room Temperature and Humidity Levels

Creating the perfect sleep environment for your baby includes paying close attention to temperature and humidity levels. The optimal room temperature for safe, comfortable baby sleep is between 68-72°F (20-22°C). This range helps regulate body temperature and prevents overheating, which can disrupt sleep and increase the risk of Sudden Infant Death Syndrome (SIDS).

Humidity also plays a crucial role in sleep quality. Maintaining a humidity level between 40-60% can prevent the air from becoming too dry or too humid, both of which can disturb a baby's sleep. Proper humidity levels help keep airways clear, reduce the risk of dry skin, and prevent congestion. Using a humidifier can be beneficial, particularly during colder months when indoor heating tends to dry out the air.

To ensure these conditions are met, use a room thermometer and a hygrometer to monitor both temperature and humidity levels consistently. Adjust your heating or cooling system, or use a fan or air conditioner, as needed to maintain the ideal environment. In dry climates or during winter, a humidifier can help keep moisture levels within the recommended range.

It's important to understand the risks associated with improper temperature and humidity. An environment that is too hot can increase the risk of overheating, which not only disrupts sleep but also raises safety concerns. On the other hand, air that is too dry can lead to respiratory issues, dry skin, and increased discomfort, causing frequent wake-ups during the night.

By carefully monitoring and adjusting these factors, you can create a safer, more comfortable sleep environment for your baby, leading to better sleep and overall well-being.

Using White Noise and Sound Machines Effectively

White noise can be a powerful tool in promoting better sleep for babies by masking disruptive background noises and creating a consistent auditory environment. This consistent sound helps soothe babies by mimicking the sounds they were used to hearing in the womb, which can make it easier for them to relax and drift into sleep.

When choosing a white noise machine, it's important to prioritize safety and effectiveness. Look for machines with adjustable volume settings so you can control the sound level. The ideal white noise machine should offer a variety of sound options—such as static, ocean waves, or rainfall—allowing you to find the sound that best suits your baby's preferences. Machines that have a timer function or an automatic shut-off feature are also beneficial to prevent continuous use throughout the night.

For effective use, ensure the machine is kept at a reasonable volume, typically around 50-60 decibels, which is roughly the volume of a normal conversation. Place the machine a safe distance from the crib—usually about 6-7 feet away—so the sound is soothing but not too overwhelming. It's also essential to avoid creating a dependence on white noise for sleep. You can gradually reduce the volume or turn off the machine once your baby is asleep to help them learn to sleep in silence over time.

For parents who prefer alternatives to dedicated white noise machines, there are many options. White noise apps on smartphones or tablets can replicate the same soothing sounds. Additionally, everyday household items like fans or air purifiers can create gentle background noise that serves a similar purpose to white noise machines.

By using white noise thoughtfully and avoiding over-reliance, you can create a calm and sleep-friendly environment that helps your baby fall asleep faster and stay asleep longer.

Safe and Comfortable Sleepwear

Choosing the right sleepwear is essential for ensuring your baby's safety and comfort during sleep. Proper sleepwear helps regulate the baby's body temperature, avoiding overheating, which is a known risk factor for SIDS (Sudden Infant Death Syndrome). Additionally, comfortable and well-fitted sleepwear minimizes the need for blankets, which can pose suffocation hazards, especially for younger infants.

When selecting sleepwear, focus on breathable materials like cotton, which allow air to circulate and keep the baby cool. Avoid synthetic fabrics like polyester, which can trap heat and increase the risk of overheating. Natural fibers are not only better for temperature regulation, but they're also soft and gentle on a baby's sensitive skin, reducing the risk of irritation.

Sleep sacks or wearable blankets are excellent alternatives to loose blankets and can keep your baby warm while maintaining a safe sleep environment. Sleep sacks come in various sizes and styles, suitable for newborns through toddlers. Look for options with adjustable sizing, allowing for room to grow while preventing the material from bunching up, which could interfere with breathing. For younger infants, opt for sleep sacks with swaddle features to promote a snug feeling similar to the womb. As your baby grows, you can transition to wearable blankets without the swaddle function, which still provide warmth without the risks associated with loose blankets.

Dressing your baby for sleep should take room temperature into account. If the room is on the cooler side (around 68°F or 20°C), consider layering with a lightweight onesie underneath the sleep sack. In warmer conditions (closer to 72°F or 22°C), a single layer of light clothing may suffice. Always check for signs of overheating by feeling the baby's chest or the back of their neck—if they're sweaty or warm to the touch, it's a sign that you may need to remove a layer. Similarly, cold hands and feet don't always indicate that the baby is too cold, but if their core feels cool, you can add an extra layer.

By dressing your baby in safe, breathable sleepwear and making adjustments based on the room's temperature, you can ensure they stay comfortable and well-regulated throughout the night.

The Benefits of Swaddling and How to Do It Right

Swaddling is a time-tested technique that can offer significant benefits for newborns. By snugly wrapping a baby in a lightweight blanket, swaddling helps create a secure and comforting environment that mimics the womb. This sense of security can calm babies, reduce anxiety, and promote longer and more restful sleep. One of the key advantages of swaddling is its ability to reduce the startle reflex (also known as the Moro reflex), which can cause babies to wake suddenly due to involuntary movements. By keeping the baby's arms snug, swaddling helps minimize these disruptions and encourages a smoother sleep cycle.

Step-by-Step Guide to Safe Swaddling:

1. **Lay out the blanket**: Spread a thin, breathable blanket on a flat surface in a diamond shape. Fold down the top corner about 6 inches to create a straight edge.

2. **Position the baby**: Lay the baby on their back on top of the blanket, with their head just above the folded edge and their body in the center.
3. **Secure the first arm**: Gently position one of the baby's arms by their side, and take the left corner of the blanket, pulling it snugly across the baby's chest, and tuck it underneath their body on the opposite side.
4. **Fold the bottom**: Fold the bottom corner of the blanket up over the baby's feet, ensuring that there's room for the baby's legs to move freely to prevent hip dysplasia. You don't want their legs tightly bound.
5. **Secure the second arm**: Gently place the other arm by the baby's side, pull the right corner of the blanket across their chest, and tuck it underneath the opposite side, leaving the baby snug but not overly tight.

Remember that swaddling should be firm enough to keep the baby feeling secure but not so tight that it restricts breathing or movement. Be sure the baby's hips can move freely, as tight swaddling around the hips can lead to hip dysplasia. Additionally, monitor the baby's temperature to avoid overheating. If they appear too warm or sweaty, adjust the swaddle or room temperature accordingly.

When to Stop Swaddling

While swaddling can be highly effective for newborns, there comes a point when it's no longer safe. Most experts recommend stopping swaddling between 2 to 3 months of age or as soon as the baby shows signs of rolling over, whichever comes first. Once a baby starts to roll, swaddling becomes a hazard, as it increases the risk of suffocation if the baby rolls onto their stomach while swaddled.

Signs that it's time to transition away from swaddling include the baby regularly breaking out of the swaddle or attempting to roll over. At this stage, you can consider transitioning to other sleep solutions that offer comfort without the need for tight wrapping.

Alternatives to Traditional Swaddling

For babies who don't respond well to traditional swaddling or for parents looking to transition away from swaddling, there are several alternatives available. Swaddle transition products, such as arms-free sleep sacks or wearable blankets, allow babies to enjoy some of the benefits of swaddling while having more freedom to move their arms and legs. Sleep suits, such as the "Merlin Magic Sleep Suit," provide a cozy yet secure environment, helping babies sleep more soundly without the risk of them rolling while tightly swaddled.

By understanding the benefits of swaddling and learning how to swaddle safely, parents can use this effective tool to promote better sleep in their newborns. Knowing when to stop swaddling and what alternatives to use ensures a smooth and safe transition as the baby grows and develops.

Managing Sleep Disruptions from External Noise

External noise can significantly disrupt a baby's sleep, making it harder for them to settle down or causing frequent wake-ups throughout the night. Understanding common sources of noise and implementing strategies to minimize these disturbances can help create a more peaceful sleep environment for babies.

Common Sources of External Noise That Disrupt Sleep:

- **Traffic sounds**: Busy streets, honking horns, or passing vehicles can create sudden and jarring noises that disrupt sleep, especially for babies sensitive to environmental changes.
- **Household noises**: Everyday sounds like conversations, the television, kitchen appliances, or footsteps can disturb a baby's sleep, particularly in smaller homes where sound travels easily.
- **Neighborhood or environmental noise**: This includes barking dogs, loud neighbors, or outdoor activities such as construction or lawnmowing, which can create inconsistent and disruptive noise levels.

Strategies for Minimizing Noise Disruptions

Creating a quieter, more insulated sleep space can make a big difference in reducing noise-related sleep disruptions.

- **Insulate windows and doors**: Using thicker or double-pane windows can help block out external traffic or neighborhood noise. Door stoppers or draft guards can also help reduce noise from other parts of the house entering the baby's room.
- **Use noise-cancelling curtains**: Heavy curtains or specialized soundproof curtains can dampen noise from outside, especially if you live in a noisy area.
- **Soft furnishings**: Rugs, upholstered furniture, and cushions can absorb sound and help reduce noise levels within the home.

By making these changes, the overall noise level in the baby's sleep space can be significantly lowered, leading to fewer disturbances during sleep.

The Role of White Noise in Masking External Sounds

White noise can be an effective tool for masking disruptive external sounds, creating a consistent auditory environment that helps babies sleep more soundly. White noise machines emit continuous, soothing sounds that mask sudden or inconsistent noises from outside the baby's room.

- **Continuous sound masking**: White noise works by creating a blanket of sound that dulls or neutralizes sudden changes in the noise environment. This helps prevent sleep disruptions caused by abrupt sounds like a barking dog or a slamming door.

To use white noise effectively, set the machine at a moderate volume, around 50-60 decibels, and place it away from the crib to avoid directly impacting the baby's hearing.

Creating a Consistent Sleep Routine

Establishing a consistent sleep routine is essential for promoting healthy sleep habits in babies. A well-structured routine not only helps signal to the baby that it's time to wind down but also builds a sense of security and predictability around sleep. Here's how to create and maintain an effective sleep routine:

The Importance of a Consistent Sleep Routine

A consistent sleep routine is beneficial for several reasons:

- **Establishing Sleep Cues**: Regular routines help condition your baby to recognize and respond to specific cues that signal it's time for sleep. These cues can include a particular sequence of activities or a specific environment that helps the baby transition from wakefulness to sleep.

- **Building a Sense of Security**: Consistency in bedtime routines fosters a sense of security and predictability, making the baby feel more comfortable and less anxious about going to sleep.

Step-by-Step Guide to Creating a Bedtime Routine

Choose Calming Activities: Select activities that help your baby relax and prepare for sleep. Typical activities include:

- **Bathing**: A warm bath can be soothing and signal the start of the bedtime routine.
- **Reading**: Reading a short, gentle story or singing lullabies can be calming and provide a transition to bedtime.
- **Feeding**: A final feeding before bed can help ensure your baby feels full and satisfied, promoting longer sleep stretches.

Establish Timing and Consistency: Aim to start the bedtime routine at the same time every night. Consistency in timing helps regulate your baby's internal clock and reinforces the sleep routine. The routine should be calm and predictable, lasting about 20-30 minutes.

Create a Relaxing Environment: Dim the lights, lower the noise levels, and use soothing sounds to create a relaxing atmosphere conducive to sleep. Ensure the sleep space is comfortable and aligned with the baby's needs.

The Role of Naps in Maintaining a Consistent Routine

Daytime naps play a crucial role in supporting nighttime sleep:

- **Coordinating Nap and Bedtime Routines**: Ensure that nap times are appropriately timed to avoid interfering with nighttime sleep. For example, a late afternoon nap might make it harder for your baby to fall asleep at bedtime. Aim for naps that are spaced out evenly throughout the day, with the last nap ending at least a few hours before bedtime.

Tips for Adjusting the Routine as the Baby Grows

As your baby grows and their sleep needs change, you may need to adjust the sleep routine:

- **Gradual Changes**: Implement changes gradually to avoid disrupting your baby's sense of security. For example, if you need to shift bedtime earlier, do so in small increments of 15 minutes over several days.
- **Monitoring the Baby's Responses**: Pay attention to how your baby responds to changes in the routine. Adjust based on their needs and feedback, such as signs of overtiredness or difficulty settling down.

By establishing and maintaining a consistent sleep routine, you help your baby develop healthy sleep habits and create a more predictable and calming sleep environment. Regular routines signal to your baby that it's time to wind down, support their overall sleep quality, and foster a sense of security and comfort around sleep.

The Role of Comfort Objects and Loveys

Comfort objects, often referred to as loveys, can play a significant role in promoting better sleep for babies. These items provide a sense of security and comfort, helping babies transition from being held by parents to sleeping independently. Here's how comfort objects can benefit sleep and how to introduce them safely:

Benefits of Comfort Objects for Sleep

- **Security and Attachment**: Comfort objects can offer a sense of security and emotional support. They become a reliable source of comfort that babies can turn to when they're feeling anxious or transitioning to sleep, helping them feel more secure and relaxed.
- **Transitioning from Parent to Object**: Loveys can assist in transitioning the baby's reliance from a parent to an object. This can be particularly helpful in fostering independent sleep, as the baby learns to soothe themselves with the comfort object rather than needing constant parental presence.

Guidelines for Introducing a Comfort Object

1. **Choose Safe, Breathable Materials**: Ensure the comfort object is made from safe, non-toxic, and breathable materials. Opt for items that are easy to clean and free from small parts that could pose choking hazards.
2. **Introduce the Object During Calm Times**: Start introducing the comfort object during calm, relaxed moments. Allow your baby to become familiar with it during playtime or while settling down rather than immediately before sleep. This helps the baby

form positive associations with the object.

Timing for Introducing Comfort Objects

- **Typically Around 6-12 Months**: Comfort objects are generally introduced when babies are developmentally ready, which is usually between 6 and 12 months of age. At this stage, babies can start to form attachments to objects and benefit from their comforting presence.
- **Developmental Signs**: Look for signs of readiness such as the ability to grasp and hold onto objects, and an increasing need for comfort and security during sleep transitions.

Suggestions for Different Types of Comfort Objects

- **Soft Toys**: Plush, soft toys that are safe for babies and easy to cuddle can serve as effective comfort objects. Ensure they are made from hypoallergenic materials and have no small parts.
- **Small Blankets**: Small, lightweight blankets or "loveys" can provide comfort and security. These should be breathable and appropriately sized to reduce any risk of suffocation.

By introducing comfort objects at the right time and ensuring they are safe and appropriate for your baby, you can enhance their ability to self-soothe and support independent sleep. Comfort objects provide a transitional source of security that can help your baby feel more comfortable and settled during sleep.

Transitioning from Co-Sleeping to Independent Sleep

Transitioning from co-sleeping to independent sleep can be a significant change for both parents and baby. This process involves moving the baby from sleeping in the same bed or room with parents to sleeping in their own crib or bed. Here's a comprehensive guide to making this transition as smooth as possible:

Benefits and Challenges of Co-Sleeping
  Benefits:

- **Enhanced Bonding**: Co-sleeping can strengthen the bond between parents and baby, providing a sense of closeness and security.
- **Ease of Night Feeding**: For breastfeeding mothers, co-sleeping can make night feedings more convenient, as the baby is readily accessible.

Challenges:

- **Risk of Transition Difficulties**: Moving the baby from co-sleeping to independent sleep may pose challenges, such as increased nighttime awakenings or resistance to change.
- **Safety Concerns**: Co-sleeping can carry risks such as suffocation or falls, which are addressed by transitioning to a separate sleep space.

Step-by-Step Guide to Transitioning to Independent Sleep

Gradual Distancing Techniques:

- **Start by Moving the Baby's Crib or Bassinet Closer to Your Bed**: Begin by placing the baby's sleep space in the same room but separate from your bed. This helps the baby adjust to sleeping in their own space while still being close to you.
- **Slowly Increase the Distance**: Gradually move the crib or bassinet further away from your bed over several nights or weeks until it is in its own room.

Establishing a New Sleep Routine:

- **Create a Consistent Bedtime Routine**: Develop a calming bedtime routine that includes activities such as a bath, reading a book, or singing a lullaby. Consistency helps signal to the baby that it's time to sleep.
- **Stick to a Regular Sleep Schedule**: Put the baby to bed at the same time each night to help establish a sense of routine and predictability.

Maintaining a Sense of Security During the Transition

- **Consistent Bedtime Routines**: Maintain the same bedtime routine to provide comfort and familiarity. This consistency can help the baby feel secure during the transition.
- **Introducing a Comfort Object**: If the baby is ready, introduce a comfort object (such as a lovey or soft toy) to provide additional reassurance and comfort in their new sleep space.

Tips for Handling Setbacks During the Transition

- **Patience and Persistence**: Understand that setbacks and resistance are normal. Be patient and consistent with the new sleep routine, and provide reassurance without reverting to old co-sleeping habits.
- **Temporary Co-Sleeping if Necessary**: If the transition proves particularly challenging, it's okay to temporarily return to co-sleeping while gradually reintroducing the independent sleep space. This should be done with the goal of eventually moving towards independent sleep.

By following these steps and maintaining a supportive and consistent approach, you can help your baby adjust to independent sleep while ensuring they continue to feel secure and comforted during the transition.

3

Gentle Sleep Training Methods

Understanding Gentle Sleep Training

Gentle sleep training is an approach that helps babies develop healthy sleep habits with minimal stress for both the child and the parents. Unlike more rigid methods, gentle sleep training emphasizes gradual changes and responsiveness to the baby's needs, aiming to foster a sense of security and trust.

What Is Gentle Sleep Training?

Gentle sleep training involves teaching your baby to fall asleep independently using methods that minimize crying and distress. The focus is on making gradual adjustments to sleep routines and behaviors, allowing the baby to adapt at their own pace. This approach respects the baby's emotional well-being and promotes a strong parent-child bond.

- **Emphasis on Minimal Crying**: Gentle methods aim to reduce or eliminate prolonged periods of crying. Parents remain close and responsive, providing comfort and reassurance as needed.

- **Focus on Gradual Changes**: Instead of abrupt shifts, gentle sleep training introduces small, manageable changes over time. This helps the baby adjust without feeling overwhelmed or anxious.

Benefits of Gentle Sleep Training

Choosing gentle sleep training methods offers several advantages over more rigid or cry-it-out approaches:

- **Reduced Stress for Both Baby and Parents**: Minimizing crying and distress makes the process less stressful for everyone involved. Parents can feel confident that they are supporting their baby's needs while working towards better sleep.
- **Promotes a Secure Attachment**: Responsive caregiving during sleep training reinforces the baby's trust in their parents. This secure attachment lays the foundation for healthy emotional development.

Addressing Common Misconceptions

There are several myths surrounding gentle sleep training that can cause confusion or doubt among parents:

- **Myth: Gentle Methods Are Not Effective**: Some believe that only strict methods yield results. However, gentle sleep training can be highly effective when implemented consistently and with patience. Many families have successfully improved their baby's sleep using gentle techniques.
- **Myth: Gentle Sleep Training Takes Too Long**: While gentle

methods may require more time than abrupt approaches, they often lead to lasting results without the stress of excessive crying. The gradual progress allows for sustainable changes that fit the baby's developmental pace.

Overview of Gentle Sleep Training Methods

There are various gentle sleep training techniques that parents can choose from, depending on their baby's temperament and the family's preferences. Here is a brief introduction to some popular methods:

- **Pick-Up/Put-Down Method**: This technique involves picking up the baby to comfort them when they cry and placing them back in the crib once they are calm. The process is repeated as needed until the baby learns to self-soothe and fall asleep independently.
- **Chair Method**: Parents sit in a chair next to the baby's crib, providing comfort through their presence. Over time, the chair is gradually moved farther away from the crib until it is eventually out of the room. This method allows the baby to adjust to sleeping alone while still feeling supported.
- **No Tears Method**: This approach focuses on eliminating crying by closely attending to the baby's needs. It involves creating a consistent bedtime routine, recognizing sleep cues, and gently guiding the baby to sleep without leaving them to cry alone.

In the following sections, we will explore each of these methods in detail, providing step-by-step guidance to help you implement the gentle sleep training technique that best suits your family's needs.

The Pick-Up/Put-Down Method

Developed by **Tracy Hogg**, known as the "Baby Whisperer," the Pick-Up/Put-Down Method is a gentle sleep training technique that emphasizes responding to your baby's needs with minimal distress. This method focuses on teaching self-soothing skills while building trust and reassurance between you and your baby.

Principles of the Pick-Up/Put-Down Method

The foundational concept of this method is to support your baby in learning how to fall asleep independently without feeling abandoned or distressed. It strikes a balance between offering comfort and encouraging self-soothing.

- **Teaching Self-Soothing**: By gradually reducing your intervention, your baby learns to calm themselves, which is essential for falling asleep independently and returning to sleep during nighttime awakenings.
- **Building Trust and Reassurance**: Consistently responding to your baby's cries establishes a sense of security. Your baby learns that you are there when needed, fostering a strong parent-child bond.

Step-by-Step Guide to Implementing the Method

1. **Prepare for Bedtime**: Establish a calming bedtime routine to signal that sleep time is approaching. This could include activities like a warm bath, gentle massage, or reading a quiet story.
2. **Place Your Baby in the Crib Awake**: After the routine, place

your baby in their crib while they are drowsy but still awake. This helps them associate their crib with the process of falling asleep.

3. **Respond to Crying by Picking Up**: If your baby begins to cry, wait a moment to see if they can self-soothe. If the crying continues or escalates, gently pick them up to offer comfort. Hold them until they are calm but not asleep.

4. **Put Down Once Calm**: Once your baby has settled, place them back in the crib. It's important to put them down before they fall asleep in your arms to reinforce their ability to fall asleep independently.

5. **Repeat as Necessary**: Be prepared to repeat the pick-up and put-down process multiple times. Patience is key, as it may take several attempts before your baby falls asleep on their own.

Appropriate Age for Using This Method

The Pick-Up/Put-Down Method is typically effective for babies aged **3 to 12 months**. Around 3 to 4 months, babies start developing the ability to self-soothe but still need parental support. This method accommodates their developmental stage by providing comfort while promoting independence.

Tips for Troubleshooting Common Issues

- **Dealing with Persistent Crying**: If your baby continues to cry despite several pick-up/put-down cycles, ensure that their basic needs are met (hunger, diaper change, discomfort). If everything seems fine, remain consistent with the method, offering calm reassurance without introducing new sleep associations.
- **Adjusting for Different Temperaments**: Every baby is unique.

Some may require longer periods of holding to calm down, while others might become overstimulated by too much picking up. Pay attention to your baby's cues and adjust the method accordingly. For instance, you might offer gentle back rubbing or soothing words instead of picking up if that seems to help more.

Success Tips

- **Stay Calm and Patient**: Your baby can sense your emotions. Remaining calm provides additional reassurance and sets a soothing tone for the bedtime routine.
- **Consistency Is Key**: Applying the method consistently helps your baby understand what to expect, which can lead to quicker adaptation and success.
- **Monitor Progress**: Keep track of how your baby responds over several nights. Small improvements, like reduced crying time or fewer pick-ups needed, indicate that the method is working.

The Pick-Up/Put-Down Method offers a compassionate approach to sleep training, allowing you to support your baby's growing independence while maintaining a strong, trusting relationship. By gently guiding them towards self-soothing, you set the foundation for healthy sleep habits that can benefit your baby well beyond infancy.

The Chair Method: Gradual Removal Technique

The Chair Method, also known as the "Sleep Lady Shuffle," was popularized by **Kim West**, a licensed clinical social worker and renowned child sleep expert affectionately known as "The Sleep Lady."

This gentle sleep training technique focuses on gradually reducing parental presence to encourage babies to develop independent sleep skills while still feeling secure and supported.

Principles and Objectives of the Chair Method

The Chair Method is designed to help your baby transition to falling asleep independently without feeling abandoned. Its main principles include:

- **Gradual Reduction of Parental Presence**: Instead of abruptly leaving your baby to sleep alone, you slowly increase the distance between yourself and your baby over time.
- **Encouraging Independent Sleep**: By offering reassurance from a distance, your baby learns to self-soothe and gains confidence in their ability to fall asleep without direct intervention.

Step-by-Step Guide to the Chair Method

Initial Stage: Sitting Beside the Crib

- **Night One**: After completing your usual bedtime routine and placing your baby in the crib drowsy but awake, sit in a chair right next to the crib.
- **Provide Reassurance**: Offer gentle words or soothing sounds to comfort your baby. You can pat or touch them if necessary, but try to minimize physical interaction.
- **Stay Until They Fall Asleep**: Remain seated until your baby drifts off. If they wake during the night, return to the chair and repeat the process.

Gradual Distancing: Moving the Chair Further Away

- **Every 3-7 Nights**: Move the chair a small distance away from the crib—perhaps a couple of feet—every few nights.
- **Maintain Presence**: Even as you move farther away, continue to offer verbal reassurance as needed. Avoid making eye contact, which can stimulate your baby.
- **Progress to the Doorway**: Continue this gradual movement until you're sitting in the doorway and eventually outside the room.
- **Final Stage: Independent Sleep**: Once you can place your baby in the crib and leave the room without them becoming distressed, they've learned to fall asleep independently.

Timeline for This Method

- **Typical Duration**: Each stage should last about **3-7 days**, but adjust according to your baby's comfort and response.
- **Signs to Advance to the Next Stage**:
- Your baby falls asleep more quickly.
- Less fussing or crying at bedtime.
- Reduced need for your verbal reassurance.

Tips for Maintaining Consistency

- **Keep a Sleep Log**: Document your baby's sleep patterns, how long it takes them to fall asleep, and any awakenings. This helps track progress and identify any patterns or issues.
- **Enlist Support from a Partner**: Sharing the responsibility can help maintain consistency and prevent burnout. Ensure that both caregivers follow the same steps and provide similar reassurance.
- **Stay Patient and Persistent**: Progress may be gradual, and

setbacks can occur. Consistency is key to helping your baby adjust to the new routine.

- **Avoid New Sleep Associations**: Be cautious not to introduce new habits like feeding or rocking to sleep during this process, as they can replace the old dependency with a new one.

By patiently implementing the Chair Method, you provide your baby with the comfort of your presence while gently encouraging them to develop the ability to self-soothe. This gradual approach respects your baby's need for security and fosters healthy, independent sleep habits over time.

The No Tears Method: Step-by-Step Guide

The No Tears Method, developed by **Dr. William Sears**, is a gentle sleep training approach rooted in the principles of attachment parenting. This method prioritizes comfort, reassurance, and responsiveness, aiming to help babies develop healthy sleep habits without experiencing distress or prolonged crying.

Philosophy of the No Tears Method

- **Emphasis on Comfort and Reassurance**: The core of the No Tears Method is to meet your baby's needs promptly and compassionately. By providing immediate comfort, whether through holding, feeding, or soothing words, you build a strong sense of security and trust with your baby.
- **Avoidance of Any Form of Crying**: This method seeks to prevent crying by proactively addressing your baby's discomfort or anxiety.

The goal is to create a peaceful sleep experience without allowing your baby to become upset or distressed.

Step-by-Step Guide to Implementing the No Tears Method

Establish a Calming Pre-Sleep Routine

- **Consistent Bedtime Rituals**: Develop a soothing routine that you follow each night. This might include a warm bath, gentle massage, soft music, or quiet reading time. Consistency helps signal to your baby that bedtime is approaching.
- **Create a Relaxing Environment**: Dim the lights and minimize noise to create a serene atmosphere conducive to sleep.

Recognize and Respond to Sleep Cues

- **Identify Signs of Sleepiness**: Look for cues like rubbing eyes, yawning, or decreased activity. Responding promptly helps prevent overtiredness, which can make it harder for your baby to fall asleep.
- **Begin the Sleep Process Early**: Start the bedtime routine at the first signs of sleepiness to ensure a smoother transition to sleep.

Provide Immediate Comfort

- **Stay Close During Sleep Initiation**: Remain near your baby as they settle down. Your presence offers reassurance and security.
- **Use Gentle Soothing Techniques**: Rocking, nursing, or gentle pats can help your baby relax. The key is to soothe them without letting them become fully dependent on these actions to fall asleep.

Gradually Reduce Parental Intervention

- **Ease Back on Soothing Over Time**: As your baby becomes more comfortable with the routine, slowly decrease the amount of intervention. For example, shorten rocking sessions or pause briefly before responding to minor fussing.
- **Encourage Self-Soothing Behaviors**: Allow your baby opportunities to settle themselves while still being available for reassurance as needed.

Maintain Nighttime Responsiveness

- **Address Night Wakings Promptly**: If your baby wakes during the night, respond quickly with comforting actions. This reinforces their sense of security and helps them return to sleep more easily.
- **Keep Interactions Low-Key**: Use soft whispers and minimal movement to avoid stimulating your baby during nighttime awakenings.

The Role of Consistency and Patience

- **Consistent Bedtime Routines**: Sticking to the same pre-sleep activities each night helps your baby know what to expect, reducing anxiety and resistance.
- **Patience with Progress**: Gentle methods may take longer to show results compared to more rigid techniques. Celebrate small victories and understand that gradual improvement is normal.
- **Regular Progress Tracking**: Keep a sleep diary to monitor patterns and improvements. This can help you adjust the approach as needed and recognize successes.

Adjusting the Method to Fit Individual Needs

- **Customizing Routines**: Adapt the bedtime routine to suit your baby's preferences and your family's schedule. What calms one baby may differ for another.
- **Flexibility in Timing**: Be willing to adjust sleep times based on your baby's signals rather than adhering to a strict clock schedule.
- **Account for Family Dynamics**: If multiple caregivers are involved, ensure everyone is consistent in applying the method to avoid confusing the baby.

Tips for Success

- **Stay Attuned to Your Baby's Needs**: Pay close attention to your baby's responses and adjust your approach accordingly.
- **Avoid Creating New Sleep Dependencies**: While providing comfort, encourage your baby to fall asleep in their sleep space rather than in your arms whenever possible.
- **Seek Support if Needed**: If you're struggling, consider reaching out to a pediatrician or a sleep consultant familiar with gentle sleep training methods.

By embracing the No Tears Method, you foster a nurturing sleep environment that honors your baby's emotional needs. This compassionate approach not only promotes better sleep but also strengthens the bond between you and your baby, laying a foundation of trust and security that supports their overall development.

Establishing a Gentle Bedtime Routine

A gentle bedtime routine is crucial for successful sleep training. It is a daily ritual that signals to your baby it's time to wind down, helping them transition smoothly from wakefulness to sleep. Consistency in this routine builds strong sleep associations, making it easier for your baby to fall asleep independently.

Importance of a Gentle Bedtime Routine

- **Signals for Winding Down**: A predictable sequence of calming activities prepares your baby's mind and body for sleep. Repetition of these cues helps them understand that bedtime is approaching.
- **Building Sleep Associations**: Consistent routines create positive associations with sleep. Over time, your baby will connect the bedtime activities with the comfort of sleeping, reducing resistance and anxiety.

Step-by-Step Guide to Creating a Bedtime Routine

Set a Consistent Bedtime: Choose a bedtime that suits your baby's age and your family schedule. Stick to this time every night to regulate their internal clock.

Begin with a Warm Bath (Optional):

- A soothing bath can relax your baby and mark the start of the bedtime routine.
- Keep the environment calm with dim lighting and gentle water play.

Dress for Sleep:

- Put on comfortable sleepwear made of breathable fabrics like cotton.
- Use a sleep sack or wearable blanket if needed for warmth.

Quiet Activities:

- **Reading**: Share a short, calming story. The sound of your voice is comforting and promotes language development.
- **Quiet Play**: Engage in low-energy activities like soft singing or looking at picture books.
- **Gentle Massage**: A light massage can relax your baby's muscles and soothe them.

Feeding:

- If part of your routine, offer a final feeding to ensure your baby is comfortable and not hungry during the night.
- Keep the feeding calm and quiet to avoid overstimulation.

Cuddle Time:

- Spend a few minutes holding, rocking, or cuddling your baby.
- Use this time for gentle whispers or lullabies to reinforce a sense of security.

Consistent Order:

- Perform these activities in the same sequence each night.
- Consistency helps your baby anticipate what comes next, easing

anxiety.

Place Your Baby in the Crib Awake:

- Lay your baby down while they are drowsy but still awake.
- This encourages self-soothing and helps them learn to fall asleep independently.

Role of Parental Involvement

- **Active Participation**: Your presence and engagement during the bedtime routine strengthen the parent-child bond.
- **Reading Stories Together**: Enhances emotional connection and provides comfort through your voice and closeness.
- **Gentle Rocking and Cuddling**: Physical touch releases oxytocin, promoting feelings of safety and affection.

Adapting the Routine as Your Baby Grows

- **Introducing New Activities**:
- Incorporate age-appropriate elements like choosing a book together or simple bedtime conversations.
- Allow your child to have a say in the routine to increase their engagement.
- **Gradual Reduction of Parental Involvement**:
- As your child becomes more independent, slowly reduce activities like rocking or lengthy cuddling.
- Encourage them to participate in tasks like dressing for bed or brushing teeth.

Tips:

- **Be Observant**: Pay attention to your baby's cues and adjust the routine to meet their changing needs.
- **Maintain Flexibility**: While consistency is key, it's okay to make slight changes to keep the routine effective and enjoyable.
- **Stay Patient**: Transitions may require time; remain patient as your baby adapts to the routine.

By establishing a gentle bedtime routine, you create a nurturing environment that promotes restful sleep. This consistent practice not only aids in successful sleep training but also fosters a deep sense of security and trust between you and your baby.

The Role of Parental Presence in Sleep Training

Parental presence is a vital component in gentle sleep training methods, offering comfort and security that ease the transition to independent sleep. Your physical and emotional availability during this process helps build trust and reassurance, which are essential for your baby's emotional development.

Significance of Parental Presence

- **Building Trust and Reassurance**: Being present with your baby as they learn to fall asleep independently reinforces their sense of safety. Your consistent presence assures them that you're there when needed, reducing anxiety and fostering a secure attachment.
- **Gradual Reduction of Dependence**: By starting with a high

level of support and slowly reducing your involvement, you help your baby adapt to sleeping on their own without feeling abruptly abandoned. This gradual approach respects your baby's emotional needs while encouraging self-soothing skills.

Strategies for Effectively Using Parental Presence

- **Sitting Beside the Crib**: Place a comfortable chair next to your baby's crib and sit with them as they settle down. Your proximity provides comfort, and your calm demeanor can help soothe them to sleep. Avoid engaging too much; instead, offer a reassuring presence.
- **Gentle Patting and Shushing**: Use soft, rhythmic pats on your baby's back or gentle shushing sounds to reassure them. This minimal intervention supports their ability to fall asleep while still feeling your comforting presence. Be careful not to overstimulate them with excessive interaction.

Gradually Reducing Parental Presence

- **Gradual Distancing Techniques**: Over several nights, slowly move your chair farther from the crib—first to the middle of the room, then near the door, and eventually outside the room. This incremental distancing helps your baby adjust to less direct support without a sudden change.
- **Monitoring the Baby's Responses**: Pay close attention to how your baby reacts at each stage. If they show increased distress, consider slowing the pace of your distancing. Your baby's comfort level should guide the progression.

Handling Separation Anxiety

- **Consistent Bedtime Routines**: Maintaining a predictable and soothing bedtime routine can alleviate separation anxiety. Familiar activities signal to your baby that it's time for sleep and that everything is as it should be.
- **Introducing Comfort Objects**: A soft toy or small blanket can serve as a transitional object, providing comfort when you're not immediately present. Ensure the item is safe for sleep—breathable, without loose parts, and appropriate for your baby's age.

Tips for Success:

- **Stay Patient and Supportive**: Separation anxiety is a normal part of development. Offering gentle reassurance without immediately picking up your baby can help them learn to self-soothe.
- **Avoid Prolonged Absences**: If your baby becomes very distressed, it's okay to offer additional comfort before resuming the gradual separation process. The goal is to reduce anxiety, not to leave your baby feeling abandoned.
- **Be Consistent**: Consistency helps your baby understand what to expect, making the transition smoother. Stick to your routine as closely as possible, even if progress seems slow.

By thoughtfully incorporating your presence into sleep training and gradually reducing it over time, you help your baby build confidence in their ability to sleep independently. This balanced approach supports healthy sleep habits while respecting your baby's need for security and comfort.

Gradual Night Weaning Techniques

Gradual night weaning is the process of slowly reducing nighttime feedings to encourage your baby to sleep for longer stretches. This gentle approach respects your baby's developmental readiness and helps them adjust without sudden changes or distress.

Understanding Gradual Night Weaning

- **Reducing Night Feedings**: Night weaning involves decreasing the number of feedings your baby has during the night. Instead of abruptly stopping, you gradually lessen feeding times or intervals, allowing your baby to adjust comfortably.
- **Promoting Longer Sleep Stretches**: As night feedings decrease, babies often begin to sleep for longer periods. This not only improves their sleep quality but also helps parents get more rest.

Why and When to Start Night Weaning:

- Most babies are ready for gradual night weaning between **6 to 12 months** of age. However, readiness can vary based on individual development and nutritional needs.
- Consult your pediatrician before beginning night weaning to ensure it's appropriate for your baby's health and growth.

Step-by-Step Guide to Gradual Night Weaning
Gradual Reduction of Feeding Duration:

- **Shorten Feeding Times**: If breastfeeding, reduce the duration of each nighttime feeding by a few minutes every couple of nights. For example, if your baby typically feeds for 10 minutes, reduce it to 8 minutes, then 6 minutes, and so on.

- **Decrease Bottle Volume**: If bottle-feeding, decrease the amount of milk or formula by small increments (e.g., reduce by 1 ounce) every few nights.

Increasing Intervals Between Feedings:

- **Extend Time Between Feedings**: Gradually increase the interval between nighttime feedings. If your baby feeds every 3 hours, try extending it to 3.5 hours for a few nights, then to 4 hours.
- **Soothing Without Feeding**: If your baby wakes up before the next scheduled feeding, use alternative soothing methods to help them return to sleep without feeding immediately.

Eliminate One Feeding at a Time:

- **Focus on Dropping the Least Necessary Feeding**: Identify which nighttime feeding your baby seems least interested in and begin by eliminating that one first.
- **Consistency Is Key**: Stick with the plan for several nights before moving on to reduce the next feeding.

Alternative Soothing Techniques

As you reduce night feedings, alternative methods can help comfort your baby:

- **Offering a Pacifier**: A pacifier can satisfy the need to suckle without feeding. Ensure it's appropriate for your baby's age and used safely.
- **Gentle Rocking or Patting**: Soothing motions like rocking or gently patting your baby's back can help them relax and fall back

asleep.

- **Soft Singing or Shushing Sounds**: Your calming voice or white noise can provide reassurance and help ease your baby back to sleep.

Handling Resistance and Setbacks

- **Staying Consistent**: Maintain your night weaning plan even if progress seems slow. Inconsistency can confuse your baby and make the process longer.
- **Offering Extra Comfort and Reassurance**: If your baby becomes upset, provide additional cuddles or soothing to reassure them without reverting to a full feeding.
- **Reassessing if Necessary**: If your baby consistently resists night weaning, consider pausing for a couple of weeks before trying again. They may not be developmentally ready yet.

Tips for Success

- **Ensure Adequate Daytime Nutrition**: Make sure your baby is feeding well during the day to reduce hunger at night.
- **Maintain a Consistent Bedtime Routine**: A predictable routine signals to your baby that it's time for a longer sleep.
- **Communicate with Caregivers**: If others assist with nighttime care, ensure everyone follows the same night weaning plan.
- **Be Patient and Flexible**: Every baby is different. Adjust the pace as needed while keeping the overall goal in mind.

By approaching night weaning gradually and with sensitivity, you support your baby's ability to sleep longer stretches while maintaining their sense of security. Remember that patience and consistency are essential, and consult your pediatrician if you have concerns or questions about the process.

Handling Sleep Disruptions During Training

Sleep training is a journey that may encounter occasional disruptions. Understanding common causes and knowing how to handle them can help you navigate these challenges without derailing your progress.

Common Causes of Sleep Disruptions

- **Illness**: When babies are unwell, their sleep patterns can be significantly affected. Symptoms like fever, congestion, or discomfort can make it difficult for them to fall asleep or stay asleep.
- **Developmental Milestones**: As babies grow, they reach milestones such as rolling over, crawling, or teething. These exciting developments can temporarily disrupt sleep due to increased brain activity or physical discomfort.

Strategies for Managing Sleep Disruptions

- **Temporary Adjustments to Routines**: Be flexible with your baby's sleep schedule during disruptions. If they're ill or going through a developmental phase, they may need extra naps or an earlier bedtime to compensate for lost sleep.
- **Extra Soothing Techniques**: Provide additional comfort to help your baby settle. This might include gentle rocking, cuddling, or soft lullabies. Sometimes, just being close can reassure them enough

to fall back asleep.

Importance of Staying Consistent

Maintaining consistency is key to successful sleep training, even when faced with disruptions.

- **Returning to the Routine as Soon as Possible**: Once the disruption has passed, gently guide your baby back to their established sleep routine. The quicker you resume consistency, the easier it will be for your baby to readjust.
- **Patience and Persistence**: Setbacks are normal. Stay patient and persistent with your approach, knowing that consistency will ultimately help your baby develop healthy sleep habits.

Tips for Preventing Future Disruptions

- **Consistent Sleep Environment**: Keep the sleep environment consistent in terms of lighting, temperature, and noise levels. Familiar surroundings provide comfort and signal to your baby that it's time to sleep.
- **Regular Sleep Schedule**: Establish and maintain a regular sleep schedule for both naps and nighttime. Predictability helps regulate your baby's internal clock and reduces the likelihood of sleep disruptions.

By anticipating potential challenges and responding with flexibility and consistency, you can minimize sleep disruptions during training. Remember that while disruptions are temporary, the healthy sleep habits you're fostering will benefit your baby for a lifetime.

Adjusting Sleep Training for Breastfed Babies

Breastfeeding offers numerous benefits for both mother and baby, but it can introduce unique challenges when it comes to sleep training. Understanding these challenges and adapting your approach can help make the process smoother while ensuring that breastfeeding continues to be a positive experience.

Unique Challenges of Sleep Training for Breastfed Babies

Frequent Night Feedings: Breastfed babies often feed more frequently than formula-fed babies because breast milk is digested more quickly. This can result in more nighttime awakenings for feedings, making sleep training a bit more complex.

Comfort Nursing: Many breastfed babies find comfort in nursing beyond just satisfying hunger. They may use nursing as a way to soothe themselves to sleep, creating a strong association between feeding and sleeping.

Strategies for Integrating Feeding with Sleep Training

Dream Feeding Techniques: A dream feed involves gently rousing your baby for a final feeding before you go to bed, typically around 10 or 11 p.m. This can help top off your baby's stomach, potentially leading to a longer stretch of sleep and reducing the need for additional night feedings.

- **How to Implement**: Gently pick up your baby without fully waking them. Offer the breast, and allow them to nurse as much as they need. Keep the environment quiet and dark to avoid overstimulation.

Gradual Reduction of Night Feedings

- **Assess Readiness**: Ensure your baby is developmentally ready to reduce night feedings, usually around 6 months, but this can vary.
- **Slowly Decrease Feeding Time**: Shorten the duration of night-time nursing sessions by a few minutes every couple of nights.
- **Increase Daytime Feedings**: Encourage more frequent feedings during the day to ensure your baby is getting enough nutrition.
- **Introduce Other Soothing Methods**: Use gentle rocking, patting, or offering a pacifier to comfort your baby back to sleep instead of immediately offering the breast.

Importance of Maintaining Milk Supply

It's crucial to ensure that sleep training doesn't negatively impact your milk production, as supply is closely linked to demand.

Monitoring Feeding Frequency and Duration:

- **Keep Track**: Use a journal or app to monitor how often and how long your baby feeds, both day and night.
- **Adjust as Needed**: If you notice a decrease in milk supply, consider adding an extra feeding during the day or expressing milk to maintain supply.

Staying Hydrated and Well-Nourished:

- **Hydration**: Drink plenty of water throughout the day to support milk production.

- **Nutrition**: Maintain a balanced diet rich in whole grains, fruits, vegetables, and lean proteins.
- **Rest**: Adequate rest can also impact milk supply, so try to rest when possible.

Involving the Partner in Sleep Training

Support from a partner can significantly improve sleep training success and help alleviate some of the pressures on a breastfeeding mother.

Taking Turns with Nighttime Soothing:

- **Alternate Responsibilities**: Partners can take over non-feeding nighttime awakenings, using soothing techniques like rocking or gentle shushing.
- **Bottle Feeding**: If the baby is accustomed to bottle feeding expressed breast milk, the partner can occasionally handle nighttime feedings.

Offering Emotional and Practical Support:

- **Encouragement**: Provide emotional support by acknowledging the challenges and being patient throughout the sleep training process.
- **Household Help**: Assist with chores or other children to allow the breastfeeding mother more time to rest and focus on maintaining milk supply.
- **Active Participation**: Engage in bedtime routines together, reinforcing consistency and showing unified support for the baby's sleep training.

By addressing the unique challenges of breastfeeding during sleep training and involving supportive strategies, you can foster better sleep habits while continuing to nurture the breastfeeding relationship. Remember that every baby is different, so it's important to remain flexible and patient as you find the approach that works best for your family.

Troubleshooting Common Sleep Training Issues

Sleep training can be a challenging process, and it's normal to encounter obstacles along the way. Understanding common issues and knowing how to address them can make the journey smoother for both you and your baby.

Common Issues During Sleep Training

Persistent Night Wakings: Despite implementing sleep training methods, some babies continue to wake frequently during the night. This can be due to various factors such as hunger, discomfort, or habitual waking.

Resistance to Bedtime Routines: Your baby may resist the bedtime routine by crying, fussing, or becoming overly active. This resistance can stem from overtiredness, overstimulation, or simply a phase of asserting independence.

Solutions for Addressing These Issues

Adjusting Sleep Schedules:

- **Reassess Nap Times**: Ensure that daytime naps are appropriately timed and of suitable duration. Too much daytime sleep or naps that are too late can affect nighttime sleep.
- **Adjust Bedtime**: If your baby is consistently resisting bedtime, consider adjusting the bedtime earlier or later by 15-30 minutes to find the optimal time when they are naturally ready for sleep.
- **Monitor Wake Windows**: Pay attention to the amount of time your baby is awake between naps and before bedtime. Adjusting these intervals can help prevent overtiredness or under-tiredness.

Reinforcing Positive Sleep Associations

- **Consistent Bedtime Routine**: Maintain a predictable sequence of calming activities before bed to signal that sleep is approaching.
- **Create a Soothing Sleep Environment**: Ensure the sleep space is conducive to rest—dark, quiet, and comfortable.
- **Use Comfort Objects**: If appropriate for your baby's age, introduce a soft toy or blanket that can provide reassurance and a sense of security.
- **Avoid Negative Sleep Associations**: Gradually reduce dependencies on feeding, rocking, or holding to fall asleep, so your baby learns to self-soothe.

Importance of Flexibility and Adaptation

Every baby is unique, and what works for one may not work for another. It's essential to be flexible and willing to adapt your approach based on your baby's responses.

Customizing Sleep Training Techniques:

- **Combine Methods**: Feel free to blend elements from different gentle sleep training methods to suit your baby's needs and your parenting style.
- **Adjust Pacing**: If progress is slow, consider taking smaller steps or allowing more time at each stage of the process.

Being Responsive to Your Baby's Cues:

- **Observe Behaviors**: Pay close attention to your baby's signals of tiredness, discomfort, or readiness for change.
- **Adapt Accordingly**: Use these observations to make informed adjustments to routines, schedules, or techniques.

Seeking Additional Support

Sometimes, despite your best efforts, challenges persist. It's important to recognize when to seek additional support.

Recognizing When to Seek Professional Advice:

- **Ongoing Sleep Problems**: If sleep issues continue for an extended period without improvement.
- **Concerns About Development**: If you suspect that sleep difficulties are affecting your baby's development or well-being.
- **Parental Stress**: If sleep challenges are causing significant stress or exhaustion for you or your family.

Finding Reputable Sleep Consultants:

- **Pediatrician Referral**: Start by discussing concerns with your pediatrician, who can rule out medical issues and may recommend a sleep specialist.

- **Credentials and Experience**: Look for certified sleep consultants with positive reviews and experience with gentle sleep training methods.
- **Aligning Philosophies**: Choose a consultant whose approach aligns with your parenting style and values.

Support Groups and Resources:

- **Parenting Groups**: Joining local or online parenting communities can provide support and practical tips from others who have faced similar challenges.
- **Educational Materials**: Books, reputable websites, and workshops can offer additional strategies and insights.

By addressing common sleep training issues with patience and flexibility, you can help your baby develop healthy sleep habits. Remember that setbacks are normal, and progress may be gradual. Stay attuned to your baby's needs, and don't hesitate to seek support when necessary. Your commitment to creating a positive sleep environment will contribute significantly to your baby's well-being and your family's overall harmony.

4

Advanced Sleep Strategies and Solutions

Dealing with Early Morning Wake-Ups

Early morning wake-ups can be challenging for both parents and babies. Understanding the reasons behind these early risings and implementing effective strategies can help extend your baby's sleep and improve everyone's morning routine.

Common Causes of Early Morning Wake-Ups

1. **Hunger**: Babies, especially younger ones, may wake up early due to hunger. Their small stomachs can only hold so much, and after several hours without feeding, they might need nourishment.
2. **Light Exposure**: Natural light signals to the brain that it's time to wake up. Early sunrise or artificial light creeping into the baby's room can trigger early wakefulness.
3. **Room Temperature**: The temperature often drops in the early morning hours. A room that's too cold or too warm can make your

baby uncomfortable, leading to early waking.

Strategies to Address and Prevent Early Wake-Ups

Adjusting Bedtime:

- **Earlier Bedtime**: Sometimes, counterintuitively, putting your baby to bed earlier can help them sleep longer. Overtiredness can lead to restless sleep and early waking.
- **Consistent Sleep Schedule**: Maintain a regular bedtime to help regulate your baby's internal clock.

Ensuring a Dark Sleep Environment:

- **Use Blackout Curtains**: Installing blackout curtains or blinds can prevent early morning light from entering the room.
- **Eliminate Light Sources**: Remove or cover any electronic devices emitting light, such as clocks or monitors.

Regulating Room Temperature:

- **Optimal Temperature**: Keep the room between 68-72°F (20-22°C) to ensure comfort throughout the night.
- **Appropriate Sleepwear**: Dress your baby in suitable clothing for the room temperature, using sleep sacks if necessary.

The Role of Bedtime Routines in Preventing Early Wake-Ups

A calming and consistent bedtime routine signals to your baby that it's time to sleep, promoting better sleep quality and potentially extending morning sleep.

Incorporating Relaxing Activities Before Bed:

- **Warm Bath**: A gentle bath can soothe your baby and help them relax.
- **Quiet Time**: Reading a story or softly singing lullabies can create a peaceful atmosphere.

Keeping Bedtime Consistent:

- **Same Time Every Night**: Putting your baby to bed at the same time reinforces their internal sleep rhythm.
- **Predictable Sequence**: Following the same steps each night helps your baby know what to expect.

Tips for Handling Early Wake-Ups When They Occur

If your baby wakes up early despite preventive measures, consider the following strategies:

Gradually Extending Wake-Up Time:

- **Delayed Response**: Wait a few minutes before attending to see if your baby resettles on their own.
- **Incremental Adjustments**: Slowly extend the time before you get your baby up, increasing by 5-10 minutes each day.

Using Quiet, Low-Stimulation Activities:

- **Keep Lights Dim**: If you need to enter the room, avoid turning on bright lights.
- **Minimal Interaction**: Provide comfort with gentle patting or

shushing, but avoid stimulating activities or play.

Avoid Reinforcing Early Waking:

- **Consistent Morning Routine**: Begin your regular morning routine at the desired wake-up time to help reset expectations.
- **Feeding Schedule**: If possible, wait until the planned wake-up time to feed, so early waking isn't associated with feeding.

Additional Considerations

- **Monitor Daytime Naps**: Ensure naps aren't too long or too late in the day, which can affect nighttime sleep.
- **White Noise Machine**: Using white noise can mask early morning sounds like birds or traffic that might wake your baby.
- **Hunger Evaluation**: For younger babies who still need night feedings, early waking due to hunger is normal. Ensure they're getting enough to eat during the day.

When to Seek Professional Advice

If early morning wake-ups persist despite trying these strategies, consider consulting a pediatrician or sleep specialist. They can help identify any underlying issues and provide tailored guidance.

By understanding the factors contributing to early morning wake-ups and implementing these strategies, you can help your baby sleep longer and start the day more rested.

Managing Multiple Night Wakings

Multiple night wakings can be challenging for both parents and babies, disrupting sleep and leaving everyone feeling fatigued. Understanding the common causes of frequent night wakings and implementing effective strategies can help minimize these interruptions and promote better sleep for your baby.

Common Reasons for Multiple Night Wakings

1. **Hunger**: For younger babies, especially those under 6 months, waking up during the night to feed is normal. Their small stomachs require frequent nourishment. However, as babies grow, they can begin to go longer stretches without needing to eat.
2. **Discomfort**: Physical discomfort is another common reason for multiple night wakings. Teething, illness, or digestive issues such as gas can cause a baby to wake up crying and uncomfortable.
3. **Sleep Associations**: Babies often develop associations with certain conditions that help them fall asleep, such as being rocked or nursed. When they wake up during the night, they might rely on these associations to fall back asleep, leading to frequent wake-ups if these conditions aren't met.

Strategies for Reducing Night Wakings

Ensuring Adequate Daytime Nutrition:

- **Balanced Feeding During the Day**: Make sure your baby is getting enough to eat during the day to reduce night hunger. This may involve more frequent feedings during the day or offering larger feedings closer to bedtime.
- **Dream Feed**: For younger babies, a dream feed before you go to bed can help top them off, potentially reducing the need for a middle-of-the-night feeding.

Addressing Sleep Associations:

- **Encourage Self-Soothing**: Gradually reduce the need for sleep associations like nursing or rocking by helping your baby learn to self-soothe. This could involve putting them down drowsy but awake, so they get used to falling asleep independently.
- **Create Positive Sleep Associations**: Use a comfort object like a small blanket or a pacifier, or create a soothing sleep environment with white noise to help your baby settle without needing constant intervention.

Monitoring Discomfort:

- **Address Teething Pain**: Use age-appropriate teething remedies if teething is disrupting your baby's sleep. Cold teething rings or a gentle gum massage can help alleviate discomfort before bed.
- **Ensure Physical Comfort**: Make sure your baby's sleep space is comfortable by regulating the room's temperature and ensuring the baby's sleepwear is appropriate.

Role of Sleep Training in Managing Night Wakings

Gentle sleep training methods can be very effective in reducing multiple night wakings by helping babies learn to sleep more independently.

1. **Gradual Night Weaning**: For older babies who no longer need to feed as frequently during the night, night weaning can help reduce night wakings. Gradually reduce the length of night feeds or increase the time between feedings to encourage longer stretches of sleep.
2. **Consistent Bedtime Routines**: Establishing a calming, pre-

dictable bedtime routine helps signal to your baby that it's time for sleep. Consistency with the routine can also help regulate their sleep cycle, reducing wake-ups during the night.

Tips for Comforting the Baby During Night Wakings

If your baby wakes up during the night, it's important to soothe them without creating negative sleep associations that can lead to more frequent wake-ups.

1. **Gentle Patting and Shushing**: If your baby wakes up, try soothing them with gentle patting or soft shushing sounds while they're still in their crib. This helps comfort them without the need to pick them up or feed them.
2. **Offering a Pacifier**: For babies who use pacifiers, offering one during night wakings can be a simple way to soothe them back to sleep without introducing a new sleep dependency.
3. **Avoid Immediate Intervention**: Give your baby a few moments to see if they can settle back to sleep on their own. Sometimes babies stir during light sleep cycles but don't necessarily need intervention unless they become distressed.

By identifying the underlying causes of multiple night wakings and applying gentle, consistent strategies, you can help your baby sleep more soundly through the night. With time and patience, both your baby and your family can enjoy more restful, uninterrupted sleep.

Strategies for Short Naps

Short naps can be frustrating for both babies and parents, as they may leave your baby feeling tired and irritable. Understanding the causes behind short naps and implementing strategies to help extend nap durations can result in more restful and restorative sleep for your baby.

Causes of Short Naps

1. **Incomplete Sleep Cycles**: Babies have shorter sleep cycles than adults, usually around 30-50 minutes. If a baby wakes up at the end of a sleep cycle and hasn't yet learned how to transition into the next cycle, this can result in short naps.
2. **External Disruptions**: Noise, light, or sudden changes in the baby's environment can easily disturb sleep, leading to wake-ups before the nap is fully restorative.
3. **Over-tiredness**: Paradoxically, being overtired can make it harder for babies to stay asleep. When babies are overtired, their bodies produce stress hormones that make it more difficult for them to fall and stay asleep, leading to shorter, less effective naps.

Strategies for Extending Nap Duration

Creating a Nap-Friendly Environment:

- **Dark Room**: Use blackout curtains to keep the room dark and mimic nighttime conditions, which can encourage longer naps.
- **White Noise**: A white noise machine or app can help drown out external sounds that may disrupt naps.
- **Comfortable Temperature**: Ensure the room is at an optimal temperature, between 68-72°F (20-22°C), so your baby is comfortable

throughout the nap.

Timing Naps Appropriately:

- **Monitor Wake Windows**: Pay attention to your baby's wake windows and schedule naps before they become overtired. As a guideline, newborns typically need a nap after 1-2 hours of awake time, while older babies may be able to stay awake for 2-3 hours.
- **Nap Duration**: For babies under 12 months, aim for at least one nap a day that is longer than an hour to ensure a deep, restorative sleep.

The Importance of Nap Routines

A consistent nap routine can help signal to your baby that it's time to sleep and improve the length and quality of their naps.

Pre-Nap Calming Activities:

- **Soothing Rituals**: Similar to a bedtime routine, pre-nap rituals like reading a book, gentle rocking, or playing calming music can help your baby wind down and prepare for sleep.
- **Consistent Cues**: Use the same calming activities before each nap to help your baby associate these cues with rest.

Consistent Nap Times:

- **Structured Nap Schedule**: Try to schedule naps at the same time each day, which helps regulate your baby's internal clock. Over time, this consistency can lead to longer, more predictable naps.

Tips for Handling Short Naps When They Occur

If your baby continues to take short naps despite efforts to extend them, it's important to remain patient and make gradual adjustments to their nap schedule.

Gradual Adjustments to Nap Timing:

- **Slightly Shift Nap Times**: If short naps persist, try adjusting the nap time by 15-30 minutes earlier or later to find the sweet spot where your baby is more likely to fall into a deeper sleep.
- **Extend Wake Time**: For babies who wake up too early from a nap, extending their wake time by 5-10 minutes before the next nap can sometimes help lengthen future naps.

Monitoring and Adjusting the Sleep Schedule:

- **Track Sleep Patterns**: Keep a log of your baby's sleep to identify patterns or triggers that might be contributing to short naps.
- **Adjust the Number of Naps**: As babies grow, they need fewer naps. If your baby is taking short naps, they may be ready to consolidate naps into fewer, longer ones. Transitioning from three naps to two, or two to one, can sometimes resolve the issue of short naps.

When Short Naps Are Normal

It's important to note that some babies naturally take short naps, particularly in the first few months. Their sleep cycles may not yet be fully consolidated, and short naps can be part of normal development. If your baby is generally content and sleeping well at night, short naps may not be a cause for concern.

By understanding the causes of short naps and implementing consistent nap routines and strategies, you can help your baby achieve longer, more restorative naps, contributing to better overall sleep and well-being.

Sleep Solutions for High-Needs Babies

High-needs babies often present unique sleep challenges due to their more intense behaviors and heightened sensitivity. Understanding what defines a high-needs baby and implementing specific strategies can help improve sleep for both the baby and the parents.

What Defines a High-Needs Baby?

High-needs babies exhibit certain characteristics that distinguish them from others, making sleep and daily routines more challenging.

- **Intense Reactions**: High-needs babies often react strongly to stimuli, whether it's hunger, discomfort, or separation from a caregiver. Their cries may be louder and more urgent, and they may become easily overwhelmed by changes in their environment.
- **Difficulty Self-Soothing**: These babies often have a harder time settling down on their own. They may rely heavily on external soothing methods, such as being held, rocked, or fed to sleep, and may resist transitioning to independent sleep.

Strategies for Managing Sleep with High-Needs Babies

Caring for a high-needs baby requires patience and a flexible approach to sleep routines. Here are some strategies that can help manage sleep challenges:

Extra Soothing Techniques:

- **Physical Comfort**: Use gentle rocking, swaddling (if age-appropriate), and cuddling to help calm your baby. Babywearing can also provide comfort during the day and help your baby feel secure.
- **Responsive Soothing**: Instead of following rigid sleep training methods, high-needs babies often respond better to a responsive approach where parents provide comfort quickly when the baby becomes distressed.

Flexible Sleep Schedules:

- **Adapt to Your Baby's Needs**: High-needs babies may not follow the same sleep patterns as other babies. Be prepared to adjust nap and bedtime schedules to fit their needs, allowing them to sleep when they show signs of tiredness rather than forcing a rigid schedule.
- **Shorter Wake Windows**: Many high-needs babies benefit from shorter wake windows, meaning they may need to nap more frequently throughout the day.

Managing Sleep During Illness

When a baby is sick, sleep can become even more challenging than usual. Illness disrupts regular sleep patterns, often leading to increased night wakings and discomfort, which can be difficult for both the baby and parents. Understanding how illness affects sleep and knowing how to manage it during these times can help everyone get through it with as much rest as possible.

Impact of Illness on Sleep

1. **Increased Night Wakings**: Illness can cause frequent night wakings due to discomfort, congestion, fever, or difficulty breathing. Babies may also wake up more often because they feel unwell and need extra comfort or attention.
2. **Discomfort and Restlessness**: Physical discomfort from symptoms like sore throats, fevers, or runny noses can make it hard for a baby to fall asleep and stay asleep. They may be more restless, frequently shifting or waking up because they feel unsettled.

Strategies for Managing Sleep During Illness

When your baby is sick, you'll need to adjust your approach to sleep in order to keep them as comfortable as possible and help them get the rest they need to recover.

Maintaining a Consistent Sleep Routine:

- **Stick to the Routine**: Even if your baby isn't feeling well, try to maintain a familiar bedtime routine. The predictability can provide a sense of comfort, helping them wind down even when they're not feeling their best.
- **Adjust the Routine**: You may need to modify the routine slightly to accommodate your baby's condition, such as skipping a bath if they have a fever, but keeping the overall structure intact is helpful.

Offering Extra Comfort and Soothing:

- **Provide Physical Comfort**: Extra cuddles, rocking, or holding may be necessary to help soothe your baby during illness. You can also use gentle back rubs or pats to provide comfort while they are in their crib.

- **Elevate the Head of the Mattress**: If your baby is congested, elevating the head of the mattress slightly can help with drainage and ease breathing. Always ensure the sleep environment remains safe.
- **Cool Mist Humidifier**: A cool mist humidifier can add moisture to the air, helping relieve congestion and making it easier for your baby to breathe, which can promote better sleep.

Importance of Monitoring and Adjusting Sleep Routines

During illness, your baby's needs will likely change, and you'll need to be responsive and flexible with their sleep schedule.

Temporary Adjustments to Sleep Schedules:

- **Extra Naps**: Illness can make babies more tired than usual, and they may need extra naps to make up for disrupted nighttime sleep. Be flexible with their nap schedule, allowing them to rest more during the day if needed.
- **Later Bedtimes**: If your baby is particularly uncomfortable or having trouble settling down, it's okay to temporarily shift their bedtime slightly to give them more time to relax.

Being Flexible and Responsive:

- **Watch for Sleep Cues**: Monitor your baby closely for signs of tiredness, such as rubbing their eyes or becoming fussy, and adjust nap or bedtime accordingly.
- **Stay Attuned to Their Needs**: Whether they need more comfort

or extra soothing techniques, remain responsive to what your baby is communicating through their behavior during illness.

Re-Establishing Sleep Routines After Illness

Once your baby starts feeling better, it's important to gradually return to their normal sleep routine. Illness can temporarily disrupt established habits, so it's essential to help your baby get back on track.

Gradual Transition Back to Normal Routine:

- **Ease Back into the Routine**: As your baby recovers, slowly transition them back into their normal bedtime and nap schedule. If you've been providing extra soothing, gradually reduce this support so your baby can return to falling asleep more independently.
- **Resume Usual Sleep Cues**: Reintroduce any pre-illness sleep cues, such as bedtime stories or lullabies, that might have been paused during sickness.

Reinforcing Positive Sleep Associations:

- **Rebuild Independence**: If your baby has become accustomed to more hands-on soothing during illness, gradually encourage them to self-soothe again by reducing the amount of physical comfort offered at night.
- **Consistency Is Key**: Stick to consistent bedtimes, naptimes, and bedtime routines to help your baby get back to a more regular sleep pattern.

By staying flexible and attentive during illness and gradually returning to your baby's regular routine afterward, you can help ensure that sleep disruptions are only temporary and your baby quickly returns to healthy, restorative sleep.

Transitioning to One Nap and Beyond

As babies grow, their sleep needs change, and transitioning from two naps to one is a significant milestone in their development. Knowing when and how to make this transition can help ensure that your baby continues to get the rest they need while adjusting to a new sleep schedule.

Signs That Indicate It's Time to Transition to One Nap

1. **Consistently Shorter Morning Naps**: One of the first signs that your baby is ready to transition to one nap is when their morning nap becomes consistently shorter, lasting less than 30-40 minutes, or they skip it altogether.
2. **Difficulty Falling Asleep for the Second Nap**: If your baby is taking longer to fall asleep for their second nap, or if the afternoon nap starts interfering with their nighttime sleep, this may be a cue that they're ready to consolidate their naps into one longer midday nap.

Other signs include increased energy in the morning or resistance to nap times that were previously predictable.

Step-by-Step Guide to the Nap Transition

Gradual Extension of Wake Times:

- **Start by Slowly Extending Morning Wake Time**: Begin by extending the time between when your baby wakes up in the morning and when they go down for their first nap. Increase wake times in 10-15 minute increments every few days until the morning nap merges into one midday nap.
- **Watch for Sleep Cues**: Pay attention to your baby's signals of tiredness, such as rubbing their eyes or becoming more fussy, and adjust accordingly. The goal is to find the right balance where they're tired enough for a longer nap but not overtired.

Adjusting Meal and Bedtime Schedules:

- **Shift Meals**: As the midday nap becomes longer, you may need to adjust your baby's eating schedule. Offer a small snack before the nap and shift lunchtime slightly earlier or later based on their new routine.
- **Move Bedtime Earlier if Needed**: During the transition, your baby may become more tired in the evening due to the longer wake time before bed. Consider moving their bedtime earlier by 15-30 minutes to compensate for the adjustment.

Impact of the Nap Transition on Nighttime Sleep

Potential for Longer Nighttime Sleep: Many babies start sleeping longer at night once they transition to one nap, as their sleep becomes more consolidated. However, some may experience temporary disruptions as they adjust to the new schedule.

Watch for Overtiredness: During the transition, your baby may show signs of being overtired, such as becoming more fussy in the late afternoon. It's important to respond by adjusting bedtime or offering a quiet, restful environment to help them wind down.

Tips for Maintaining a Consistent Nap and Bedtime Routine

Consistent Nap Timing: Once your baby has settled into one nap, try to keep it at the same time every day, typically after lunch. This helps regulate their internal clock and makes it easier to predict when they'll need sleep.

Establish a Pre-Nap Routine: Just like with bedtime, a calming pre-nap routine can help signal to your baby that it's time for sleep. This could include reading a short book, singing a lullaby, or a few minutes of quiet play.

Stick to Bedtime Routines: Keep your bedtime routine consistent to ensure that nighttime sleep remains stable during the nap transition. Familiar activities like a warm bath, reading, or gentle rocking help your baby relax and prepare for bed.

By paying attention to your baby's cues and following a gradual, flexible approach, you can make the transition to one nap as smooth as possible. With the right balance of sleep and a consistent routine, your baby can continue to get the rest they need for healthy growth and development.

5

Parental Well-Being and Support

The Importance of Parental Sleep and Well-Being

As much as sleep is crucial for babies, it's equally important for parents. When parents are well-rested, they are better equipped to care for their baby, make sound decisions, and manage the demands of daily life. Adequate sleep plays a significant role in maintaining both physical and mental health, enhancing emotional regulation, and supporting overall well-being.

Why Parental Sleep is Crucial

1. **Improved Cognitive Function and Decision-Making**: When parents are well-rested, they are more alert and capable of making better decisions. Sleep helps improve memory, focus, and problem-solving abilities—skills essential for navigating the complexities of parenting.

2. **Enhanced Emotional Regulation**: Adequate sleep allows parents

to manage their emotions more effectively, leading to increased patience, resilience, and the ability to remain calm in challenging situations. It also helps reduce stress, making it easier to balance the demands of parenthood.

Effects of Sleep Deprivation on Parenting

1. **Increased Irritability and Impatience**: Sleep deprivation can make parents more irritable, less patient, and quicker to react emotionally. This can lead to frustration in managing daily tasks and negatively affect interactions with both the baby and other family members.
2. **Higher Risk of Postpartum Depression**: Persistent lack of sleep has been linked to a higher risk of postpartum depression and anxiety. Sleep deprivation exacerbates feelings of helplessness or overwhelm, making it harder to manage the emotional challenges of early parenthood.

Strategies for Improving Parental Sleep

1. **Napping When the Baby Naps**: One of the simplest yet most effective ways for parents to catch up on rest is to sleep when the baby sleeps. Even short naps during the day can help parents recharge and reduce the effects of sleep deprivation.
2. **Sharing Nighttime Duties with a Partner**: Dividing nighttime responsibilities can make a significant difference in both parents getting more rest. Taking turns feeding, changing, or soothing the baby helps distribute the workload, ensuring that both parents have opportunities for uninterrupted sleep.
3. **Creating a Sleep-Friendly Environment**: Just like babies, parents can benefit from creating an environment conducive to

sleep. This includes a dark, quiet room, a comfortable mattress, and minimizing screen time before bed to ensure more restful sleep.

The Importance of Self-Care Routines

1. **Regular Physical Activity**: Exercise is a natural stress reliever and energy booster. Even a short walk or yoga session can help parents feel more energized during the day and improve the quality of their sleep at night.
2. **Mindfulness and Relaxation Techniques**: Mindfulness practices such as meditation or deep breathing exercises can help reduce stress and promote relaxation. Taking a few moments to practice mindfulness can make it easier for parents to fall asleep and stay asleep, even during busy or stressful times.

By prioritizing sleep and self-care, parents can enhance their well-being, build emotional resilience, and ensure they have the energy needed to care for their baby. Small changes to daily routines and nighttime habits can lead to significant improvements in both parental health and family dynamics.

Using Sleep Logs and Tracking Progress

Sleep logs can be a valuable tool for parents to better understand and improve their baby's sleep patterns. By tracking and analyzing sleep data, parents can identify trends, monitor progress, and make informed decisions to create a more consistent and effective sleep routine.

Benefits of Using Sleep Logs

1. **Identifying Patterns and Trends**: A sleep log provides insight into your baby's natural sleep rhythms. By documenting sleep times, naps, and night wakings, parents can recognize patterns that may not be immediately obvious. This helps to identify whether certain factors, such as late naps or feeding times, are affecting nighttime sleep.

2. **Monitoring Progress Over Time**: Tracking sleep allows parents to see how their baby's sleep evolves over days or weeks. Whether you're implementing a new sleep routine or navigating sleep challenges, a sleep log helps measure progress, allowing you to adjust as needed.

Guidelines for Maintaining a Sleep Log

Tracking Sleep Duration and Wake Times:

- Record the start and end times of naps and nighttime sleep.
- Note the duration of each nap and any nighttime wake-ups to understand how long your baby is sleeping overall.

Noting Feeding and Nap Times:

- Track feeding times, especially if your baby is still feeding at night. This can help identify whether night wakings are hunger-related or habitual.
- Include nap times to see how daytime sleep affects nighttime rest and whether nap lengths or schedules need adjustment.

Capturing Mood and Behavior:

- Consider noting your baby's mood upon waking, as this can indicate how restful their sleep was. A well-rested baby is typically happier and more alert, while frequent wake-ups may lead to crankiness.

Encouraging Patience and Persistence

Sleep training is a process that requires patience, persistence, and a positive mindset. There will be gradual progress, setbacks, and moments of frustration, but maintaining a calm and consistent approach is key to achieving long-term success in helping your baby develop healthy sleep habits.

The Importance of Patience in Sleep Training

1. **Gradual Progress and Setbacks**: Sleep training is not a quick fix. Progress often comes in small, gradual steps, and occasional setbacks are normal. Understanding that sleep habits develop over time helps parents remain patient and focused on the bigger picture.

2. **Building Trust and Security**: Patience in sleep training fosters a sense of trust and security between parents and their baby. By responding consistently and gently to their baby's needs, parents help build the foundation for long-term sleep success without causing undue stress or anxiety.

Strategies for Maintaining Persistence

Setting Realistic Goals:

- Break down sleep training goals into small, achievable steps. Rather than expecting a full night's sleep right away, aim for milestones like reducing the number of night wakings or extending naps by 10-15 minutes.

- Remember that each baby is unique, and progress may happen at a different pace. Set goals that reflect your baby's developmental stage and temperament.

Celebrating Small Successes:

- Recognize and celebrate small victories, such as your baby falling asleep more quickly or sleeping a little longer than usual. These small wins are signs that progress is being made, even if the overall journey feels slow.
- Reward yourself and acknowledge the effort you're putting into sleep training. Positive reinforcement helps keep your motivation high.

The Role of a Positive Mindset

Focusing on Progress Rather than Perfection:

- Rather than aiming for a perfect outcome, focus on the incremental progress being made. Babies' sleep patterns evolve, and focusing on improvements rather than perfection can help you stay motivated.
- Remind yourself that sleep training is a process, and it's okay if things don't go perfectly every night. A positive mindset will help you navigate challenges with resilience.

Practicing Self-Compassion:

- It's natural to feel frustrated or discouraged at times, but practicing self-compassion is essential. Be kind to yourself, acknowledge the challenges you're facing, and avoid self-criticism.

- Remember that sleep training takes time, and all parents experience ups and downs. Give yourself grace and recognize the effort you're putting into caring for your baby.

Tips for Staying Motivated

Seeking Support from Partners and Friends:

- Reach out to your partner, friends, or family for emotional support and encouragement. Sharing the experience with others can help lighten the load and remind you that you're not alone in this journey.
- Consider connecting with other parents who are going through similar sleep challenges. Parenting communities, both online and in-person, can provide valuable advice and motivation.

Reminding Yourself of the Long-Term Benefits:

- Keep the long-term benefits of healthy sleep in mind. The short-term challenges of sleep training are outweighed by the long-term advantages of better sleep for both you and your baby, including improved well-being, mood, and energy levels.
- Visualize the eventual outcome of consistent sleep for your family, and use that as motivation during difficult times.

By embracing patience, maintaining persistence, and cultivating a positive mindset, parents can successfully navigate the challenges of sleep training. Staying motivated and recognizing the importance of self-care and support ensures that both parents and baby benefit from the process in the long run.

6

Conclusion

T his book was created with one clear vision in mind: to empower parents with the knowledge, tools, and strategies to navigate the complex world of baby sleep. Understanding baby sleep is not only essential for your child's development and well-being but also for your own mental and physical health. By providing gentle, actionable approaches to sleep training, we aimed to support your journey in building healthy, sustainable sleep habits for both your baby and your family.

Recap of Key Points from Each Chapter

1. **Understanding Baby Sleep**: We explored the fundamentals of baby sleep, including the different stages of sleep and how they evolve as your baby grows. By understanding these cycles, you can better anticipate and manage your baby's sleep needs.
2. **Creating a Sleep-Friendly Environment**: We discussed the importance of setting up a conducive sleep space, covering everything from safe sleep practices to the role of light, temperature, and sleepwear. A comfortable and safe sleep environment lays the

foundation for better rest.

3. **Gentle Sleep Training Methods**: In this chapter, we offered a variety of gentle approaches to sleep training, including the Pick-Up/Put-Down Method, the Chair Method, and the No Tears Method. Each technique emphasized minimal crying, patience, and supporting your baby's natural development.

4. **Advanced Sleep Strategies and Solutions**: Here, we tackled more specific challenges, such as early morning wake-ups, managing night wakings, and addressing sleep disruptions due to illness or developmental changes. Tailored strategies help you adapt to your baby's evolving sleep needs.

5. **Parental Well-Being and Support**: Finally, we focused on the importance of parental sleep and self-care. We emphasized the need for parents to maintain their own well-being through sleep, self-care routines, and shared responsibilities. Parenting is a challenging journey, and taking care of yourself is crucial to being the best version of yourself for your baby.

Key Takeaways

- **Consistency and Flexibility**: Consistency is key in setting routines, but flexibility is equally important. Babies grow and change rapidly, and their sleep needs evolve with time. Learning to adapt without losing sight of the routine helps maintain balance.

- **Gentle Sleep Training**: There's no one-size-fits-all solution for sleep training. The gentle methods outlined in this book offer options that respect your baby's emotional needs and help build trust and security while guiding them toward independent sleep.

- **Parental Self-Care**: Healthy sleep habits for your baby also depend on your well-being. Make sleep and self-care a priority for yourself, and seek support when needed to avoid burnout and exhaustion.

As parents, it's natural to want quick results, but sleep training is a process that takes time and effort. Set realistic expectations for yourself and your baby, and remember that progress isn't always linear. There will be setbacks, growth spurts, and illnesses that disrupt the process, but with patience, persistence, and flexibility, you'll see improvements.

Now that you're equipped with the tools and knowledge to navigate baby sleep, the next step is to put these strategies into action. Start by observing your baby's sleep patterns, implementing gentle sleep training methods, and creating a supportive sleep environment. Every small step you take brings your family closer to healthier, more restful sleep.

Parenthood is a journey filled with both challenges and joy. Sleep, though seemingly a small aspect, is foundational to the well-being of your baby and your family. By staying patient, flexible, and compassionate with yourself and your child, you are already doing an amazing job. Trust the process, trust your instincts, and remember— you've got this. You are capable, resilient, and fully equipped to handle whatever comes your way.

Rest easy, knowing that better sleep is within reach. Your family's well-being is worth every effort, and together, you will find the balance and peace you need for the journey ahead.

7

Resources

Hogg, T., & Blau, M. (2005). The baby whisperer solves all your problems (by teaching you how to ask the right questions): sleeping, feeding, and behavior - beyond the basics from infancy through toddlerhood. In *Vermilion eBooks*. http://ci.nii.ac.jp/nc id/BA88830979

Msw, K. W. (2023). *The Sleep Lady®'s gentle newborn sleep guide: Trusted Solutions for Getting You and Your Baby FAST to Sleep Without Leaving Them to Cry It Out*. BenBella Books.

Sears, W., Sears, J., Sears, M., & Sears, R. (2014b). *The Baby Sleep Book: The Complete Guide to a Good Night's Rest for the Whole Family*. Little Brown.